Hormone Heresy

What Women Must Know About Their Hormones

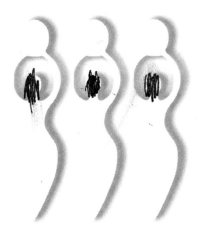

DR. SHERRILL SELLMAN, ND

1st Edition: March 1998

2nd Edition: June 1999

3rd Edition: October 2000

4th Edition: September 2001

ISBN: 978-0-9799176-7-7

Published By:

Bridger House Publishers, Inc.

PO Box 599, Hayden ID, 83835

1-800-729-4131

Cover graphics: G3&Duck Designs

Typesetting: Julie Melton, The Right Type, USA therighttype.com

Printed in the United States of America

Contents

Foreword xiii

Acknowledgements xv

Introduction xvii

PART ONE

The Untold Hormone Story

Chapter 1

Getting the Story Straight 1
The Waning of Women's Health and Power 2
The History of Hormone Replacement............................. 5
Another Perspective 7

Chapter 2

A Brief Gynecological Tour of a Woman's Body............................ 11

Chapter 3

The Myth of Synthetic Estrogen and Progestins 19

Chapter 4

A Lesson from History 23
Dishonest Beginnings... 24
The Truth Comes to Light 24

Chapter 5

Introducing Estrogen Dominance 27
Growing Hormonal Imbalances 29
Female Health Problems on the Rise............................... 30
Perimenopause 32
Symptoms of Estrogen Dominance 34
Effects of Estrogen Dominance 36

Chapter 6

Adding Still Another Ingredient to the Hormone Soup 39
Potential Side Effects of Medroxyprogesterone Acetate 40

Chapter 7

And the Synthetic Hormones Just Keep Coming 45

Chapter 8

Hormone Addiction 48

Chapter 9

Estrogen Dominance in the Environment 49
Disturbing Changes 50
The Israeli Breast Cancer Finding 51
What the Future Portends 52

Chapter 10

The Myth of Estrogen Deficiency 55

Chapter 11

But My Blood Tests Say 59
Blood Spot Testing 60
What's the Skinny on Bio-Identical Hormones 61

Chapter 12

The Pill—A Bitter Pill to Swallow 63
Minor Side-effects of the Pill 69
Major Side-effects of the Pill 70

Chapter 13

Enter Natural Progesterone 71
PMS Is Real 72
Progesterone Remembered 72
A Recurring Theme 74
Functions of Progesterone 76

Chapter 14

Discovering Some of the Benefits of Natural Progesterone.........77
Aches and Pains of the Muscles (Fibromyalgia)............................78
Allergies...78
Arthritis 78
Auto Immune Disorders 79
Candida..79
Endometriosis..79
Fibroids 81
Hair Loss and Increased Facial Hair..82
High Blood Pressure 82
Hot Flashes..83
Infertility, Early Miscarriages and Post Natal Depression..........84
Migraine Headaches...86
Ovarian Cysts 86
Premenstrual Syndrome..87
Sex Drive (Low Libido) 88
Skin Problems...89
Thyroid Deficiency 89
Vaginitis, Vaginal Dryness and Thinning 90

Chapter 15

Suggested Uses of Natural Progesterone 93
How to Apply It?..94
When to Use It? 94
Hormone Replacement Therapy — How to Get Off It.................94
Hysterectomies...96
Menopause...98
Osteoporosis 99
Perimenopause 99
PMS 101

Chapter 16

Natural Estrogens — The Good Guys...103
Estriol — The Underestimated Estrogen 104

Chapter 17

The Relationship between Hormonal Imbalance and Disease.. 107
Exposing the Myths 107
Osteoporosis 107
Cardiovascular Disease... 112
Hormones and Cancer... 117
Breast Cancer 117
Tamoxifen — Beware 119
Endometrial Cancer 121
Cervical Cancer... 121
Ovarian Cancer.. 121
Melanomas.. 122
Alzheimer's Disease 122

Chapter 18

Men and Natural Progesterone 125

Chapter 19

An Integrative Approach 129

Chapter 20

The Challenge Before Us.. 131

PART TWO

The Journey to Hell and Back
Women's Personal Stories

A Personal Perspective 136
Katie's Story 137
Franka's Story 140
Terri's Story.. 143
Linda's Story 146
Sally's Story.. 148

PART THREE

The Feminine Path to Power

Chapter 1
Looking into the Crystal Ball..155

Chapter 2
Forgotten History 157
The Feminine is Forgotten...158
The Awakening...159
Lunar Consciousness..161
The Truth about Menopause 162
Creating Sacred Feminine Power 164

Chapter 3
Women's Power and Women's Health Choices..........................167
A New Understanding of the Mind/Body.................................168

PART FOUR

Returning to Balance

Chapter 1
Walking the Middle Path 173

Chapter 2
Food is Medicine..175
Bioflavonoids 176
Boron 176
Phytohormones 176
Essential Fatty Acids (EFAs)..177

Chapter 3

Foods to Avoid..179
    Refined Sugar 179
    Caffeine...179
    Processed Oils..179
    Refined Flours and Grains 180
    Dairy Products...180
A Word about Vitamins...181

Chapter 4

Precious Water 183

Chapter 5

The Breath of Life 185
The Healing Breath 186

Chapter 6

Use It or Lose It...187

Chapter 7

Meditation—Moving Inwards 189

Chapter 8

Loving Your Body 191

Chapter 9

Emotional Healing and Spiritual Growth 193

Chapter 10

Coming Full Circle...195

PART FIVE — Updated Section

How to Get Younger and Healthier as We Get Older

Chapter 1

Getting Younger and Healthier As We Get Older 199

Chapter 2

The Physiology of Hormones 203
Digestion, Malabsorption and Candida 204
A Rise in Hypothyroidism 206
The Adrenal Glands 208

Chapter 3

How to Balance Your Menopausal Moods 211
Hormonal Imbalance 212
Avoid Steroids 212
Correct Underlying Problem 213

Chapter 4

Natural Solutions for Healing Uterine Fibroids 215
Fibroids and Hormonal Imbalance 215
Balance Hormones, Banish Fibroids 216
Fibroids and Your Liver 217
The Benefits of Castor Oil Packs and Coffee Enemas 218
Coffee Enema Recipe 220
The Thyroid — Fibroid Connection 220
Other Useful Strategies 221

Chapter 5

Hysterectomies — A Surgical Assault of Women 223
What is a Hysterectomy? 224
Why Have One? 225
The Side-effects 225
What Women Aren't Being Told 226
Regaining Control Over Our Bodies 227
Facts About A Hysterectomy 229

Chapter 6

Osteoporosis: The Bones of Contention............................231
The Bare Bones About Bones..232
The Bone-Building Drug Scam...235
Building Healthy Bones 236

Chapter 7

The Ancient Secret for Hormonal Balance........................239
The Pomegranate, A Woman's Elixir................................240
The Pomegranate, Hormones and Menopause 241
Pomegranate and Breast Health 243
Pomegranate for Vaginal Health......................................244
Vaginal Dryness Progam...245
Pomegranate Seed Oil for Healthy, Glowing Skin 246
Back to the Future with Pomegranate Fruit.......................246

Chapter 8

The Antidote to Being Frazzled and Foggy 247
L-theanine to the Rescue 248
Suntheanine Helps..250

Chapter 9

What's Up with this Weight Gain?....................................253
Enter the Ultimate Fat Loss and Body Resculpting Program....254
The Thyroid Is Not the Answer 256
Dr. Simeons' Gift to an Overweighted World.....................257

Chapter 10

Let Food Be Your Medicine...261
The Return of the Super-Seed...262
A World of Nutrition in a Tiny Seed.................................262
Women's Health and Salba...264
The Healing Power for Diabetes & Metabolic Syndrome 265
A World of Nutrition for Us All 266

Chapter 11

Super Charge Your Immune System 269
Our Intelligent Immune System 270
PeakImmune4 – A Biological Response Modulator to the Rescue... 271
A Life Saving Supplement 272
A Strong Immune System is Your Best Health Insurance 274

Chapter 12

Glutathione — The Miracle Molecule for Longevity 275
The Life-Extending Master Antioxidant 276
Essential Support of Immunity and Detoxification 277
Glutathione's Role in Cancer Prevention 278
The Miracle Molecule 279
Increasing Glutathione Levels 279

Chapter 13

Drugs on Tap 283
Would You Like Birth Control Pills With Your Coffee? 284
Antibiotics — Too Much of A Good Thing 285
Just Drink Your Prozac and Call Me in the Morning 286

Chapter 14

The Total Body Detox Solution 289
One More Piece to the Toxicity Puzzle 290
Zeolite — Removes Toxins Naturally 291
A Silver Lining Against Pathogens 292
The Total Body Detox Solution 293
Total Silver — A Dynamic Duo 294
Cleanse and Live Vibrantly! 295

Chapter 15

The Wireless Dilemma:
    Hormones Disruption, Breast Cancer and Cell Phones 297
Anatomy of Electropollution 101 298
Hormones, Cell Phones and Electropollution 298
More Hormone Disruption 301
Cortisol, Stress and What's in the Airways 302
Three Pieces of the Intervention Puzzle 303

Chapter 16

Practical Protocols for Women's Health 305
    Hormone Wreckers 305
    Hormone Harmonizers 306
Recommended Nutritional Protocols............................. 307
    Breast Cancer Prevention.. 307
    Candida Yeast Infections.. 308
    Detoxification Support 308
    Endometriosis... 309
    Fibrocystic Breast Disease... 309
    Fibroids... 310
    Heart Disease Prevention 310
    Osteoporosis 311
    Ovarian Cysts 312
    Perimenopause and Menopause Support 312
    Polycystic Ovarian Syndrome (PCOS).................... 313
    Premenstrual Syndrome 314
    Skin Problems.. 315
    Stress, Anxiety Attacks and Night Sweats 315
    Vaginal Dryness and Atrophy.................................. 316

Chapter 17

Resources for Hormonal Balance and Optimal Health 317

Chapter 18

Educational and Support Resources 335

References... 337

About the Author 343

Index 345

Foreword:

When Dr. Sherrill Sellman and I met over ten years ago, we shared what has been called a mutual resonance, a feeling of total bonding and synchronous harmonies, as if we were beloved sisters, which, of course, in the great cosmic picture, we are.

Hormone Heresy: What Women MUST Know About Their Hormones is a courageous, yet balanced book: it dances us through the history of how women and their powerful hormones have been so carelessly rendered by the medical-pharmaceutical-industrial complex, so aptly named by our mentor, John R. Lee, MD. It reminds us, happily, that if we treat our bodies, minds, and souls with utmost love, respect, and compassion, we can journey from the maiden years to the crone years with our beauty, our sensuality, and our wisdom firmly intact.

Sherrill's wonderful teachings, through her book, her website, and her interviews all speak of her great passion for illuminating and empowering her followers. And she does it with integrity, love and grace.

Helene B. Leonetti MD
Obstetrics and Gynecology
Lehigh Valley Health Network
Bethlehem, PA

Author:
Hardwired for Love: Nurturing Yourself to Vibrant Health

Acknowledgements

My gratitude to my parents,
Ruth and Harry,
who nurtured my tender spirit
with love.

My gratitude to my dearest friend, James,
who always believed in me,
even when I didn't.

My gratitude to the women
throughout the world
who are following
their inner wisdom,
reclaiming their power,
speaking their truth and
giving birth to a new world.

Introduction

As I fulfil my vision of writing this book, I am driven by my passion to share with women of all ages a greater understanding of their hormonal nature and the safe alternatives that are presently available. I often posed the question to myself, "Who am I to write this book?" As one woman in search of her truth, I realized that truth does not exclusively lie in the domain of the intellectuals or the professionals (often they are the ones most blinded by vested interests) nor in hallowed academic classrooms nor scientific laboratories. Like so many other women who are now awakening to their wise woman within, I am being guided by my intuitive wisdom not only to fulfil a greater purpose but also to speak my truth. As guardians of the sacred gift of Life, it is time for all women to courageously share their wisdom and speak up for what they believe.

My search began when it suddenly dawned upon me one day that I was rapidly approaching my menopausal years. I really hadn't thought very much about menopause—it seemed like I had years to go before I would have to deal with that mysterious 'change of life'. But changes were beginning to happen to my body—night sweats, low libido, periods of anxiety and depression, a few new hairy recruits to my face and sometimes irregular periods with clotting. I really knew nothing about this unspoken milestone in a woman's life. Was I supposed to dread the inevitable or rejoice in its arrival? I didn't have much information to go on. I certainly don't remember my mother having said a thing to me about her experience of menopause. It was as mysterious to me as my first initiation into womanhood— menstruation. At that time, I didn't know much about the workings of my body. And, in all honesty, I must admit that at forty-four years of age the physiology of the female body was still rather a mystery to me.

Thus, I began my exploration into the realm of menopause. I thought the exercise would be to simply learn the facts and, ultimately, to make an informed decision about Hormone Replacement Therapy. It turned out to be so much more. The curiosity which led me on this journey catapulted me into unexpected domains. Like Alice walking through the looking glass, I ventured into a topsy-turvy world where nothing was as it appeared to be. What was presented as truth upon closer scrutiny dissolved into illusion.

The more I explored this subject, the more I stumbled upon an entangled maze of myths, misinformation and propaganda. I discovered that the treatments of medical science for managing women's hormonal problems were fraught with many unseen dangers. While many of these treatments are proclaimed as either perfectly safe or having only minimal risks or side-effects, in actuality there is nothing safe about pharmaceutically or surgically tampering with women's hormones.

My continuing research caused me to challenge the most sacrosanct belief about the menopausal woman—that she is estrogen deficient. It was becoming apparent that 'estrogen deficiency' was a completely erroneous assumption. At first I could hardly believe what I was discovering. What about the millions of women around the world who are presently receiving synthetic or bio-identical hormones to correct their supposed 'estrogen deficiency'? Could it really be that all these women are being misdiagnosed? Could it be that the medical profession, spurred on by the billion dollar pharmaceutical industry, was way off track? The simple answer is yes. The complex answer, however, requires delving much more deeply into a myriad of political, cultural and economic issues as well as conflicting paradigms.

As I sought out the researchers, medical doctors and writers who helped me to bring this picture into focus, the true story began to emerge. It involves not just the issue of menopause but the wide-scale use of synthetic estrogen and progestins (which is synthetic progesterone) to treat women at all ages of their life—from their teenage years right through to their post-menopausal years. The following chapters will provide a totally different perspective on the hormone story than has previously been available to most women and, for that matter most health practitioners. I have written this book in simple language so that every woman (and man) can easily understand the issues at hand and the risks at stake.

But there is much more to this story. It involves a greater awareness of what is happening to our environment through the toxic estrogenic pollution from the indiscriminate use of herbicides, pesticides and plastics over the last four decades and the serious effects such changes have upon our hormonal health. It necessitates a reappraisal of our life-style—illustrating the importance and necessity of clean air, pure water and organic foods.

This story also concerns each woman's personal journey of empowerment and the honoring of her own intuitive wisdom. It's about women regaining responsibility for their own bodies and returning to a greater connection to natural cycles. Regaining this balance is crucial for the survival of our planet! It is, also intimately linked to finding the balance within oneself physically, emotionally, mentally and spiritually.

As is so often the case, embarking upon this journey has profoundly transformed me. My personal quest for most of my life has been to find within myself a deep sense of inner peace, confidence, self-acceptance and courage to express my creative gifts. It has been a long and often painful process with many recurring bouts of feeling inadequate and powerless.

Like so many other women, I was in a constant battle with my body, regularly assaulting it with diets, food fads, deprivation and disdain. These inner stresses would frequently manifest as allergies, irregular periods, fatigue, PMS, anxiety attacks and depression.

What began as curiosity about the changes occurring in my body gained momentum to become a quest for knowledge. Through the years I investigated natural alternatives to balance my hormones with dietary changes, herbs, meditation and exercise. Part of my personal quest was to reclaim my appreciation for being a woman. I realized that menstrual cycles expressed not only physical changes in my body but also psychological and spiritual changes—a part of the mystery of being female I never understood before. I began to listen more closely to my intuition and the needs of my body, emotions and spirit. I've now come to realize how truly miraculous it is to be a woman.

As I integrated this new awareness and these new behaviors, my life began to change. My body began to heal and eventually all my physical symptoms totally disappeared. Even those symptoms which I thought were the inevitable signs of menopause were more about the stress and disharmony within me than actual menopause. My health is now the best it has ever been. To my great delight I have also discovered a growing sense of well-being. I am no longer feeling afraid and insecure. As I continued to honor myself and my emotional and physical needs, I feel more centered within. I have at last arrived at a time of my life when I can honestly say I love who I am—a major accomplishment from those old days of self-hatred.

With each passing day I find myself tapping into a more profound and personal understanding of feminine power. I have come to realize that for a woman to truly reclaim her true power, she must embody a deep appreciation and reverence for herself as an expression of the Feminine. It is a multi-faceted journey. Coming into hormonal balance requires a rebalancing and aligning on all levels. After all, our bodies are an expression of what we feed them—through our thoughts, our emotions, our diet, our actions and our creative expression. I have included in this book further information and practical strategies which I have personally experienced and from which I have benefited for creating this greater inner and outer balance.

By having the courage to explore, to question and even to challenge the status quo within myself as well as in the outer world, I am at last awakening to the power of my Feminine Self. Life is a most joyful and wondrous adventure for me now. And my wish is that as you read this book, you too will be inspired to begin your journey to greater health and feminine wisdom.

Hormone Heresy

PART ONE
The Untold Hormone Story

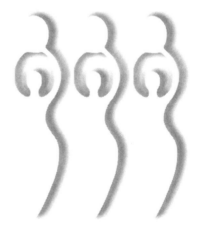

Chapter 1

Getting the Story Straight

Synthetic hormones, in the form of estrogen or progestins, are quite high profile these days. For some they represent the Golden Fleece that excites so many medical practitioners, pharmaceutical companies and writers in search of their miraculous properties. For others, estrogen and progestin are rather perilous hormones, fraught with many unknown and unspoken dangers. Most women are lost in the dark and bottomless abyss, somewhere between truth and fiction. All to often they are desperately confused about whether to trust their instincts or medical science. Nothing less than their physical, emotional and mental health and long term well-being hang in the balance.

This hormone story is similar to a modern day thriller. It is a story of deception, betrayal, hidden agendas, propaganda and misinformation. As a story it could be quite entertaining but as a real life drama its effects are disastrous to the lives of tens of millions of women around the world.

Hormones are very powerful substances. Begin tampering with nature's finely tuned messengers of life's processes and you are asking for trouble. This is especially true for women. A woman's psyche is intimately connected to her monthly flow of hormones. Hormones not only direct and determine her physiological processes but also influence her emotional and psychological state. Besides creating a myriad of health problems and diseases, hormonal imbalance can undermine self-esteem, creativity, mental acuity and a healthy sex drive.

Perhaps the bigger picture about the hormone story lies in the fact that the introduction of synthetic hormones, as a purportedly legitimate need of women, is basically experimentation under the guise of standard medical practice. As a result, medical science has expanded its control over women's lives. A sense of powerlessness and hopelessness seem to permeate a woman's existence.

Germaine Greer, well-known feminist and author of *The Change*, sums up the medical establishment's intrusion into a woman's hormonal health quite astutely when she says, "Menopause is a dream speciality for the mediocre medic. It requires no surgical or diagnostic skill, it is not itself a life-threatening condition, there is no scope for malpractice action. Patients must return again and again for a battery of tests and check-ups."[1]

> *Quite simply, tampering with*
> *a woman's hormones*
> *is tampering with her power.*

The Waning of Women's Health and Power

For over three hundred years, beginning in the thirteenth century and continuing well into the sixteenth century, the Inquisition was a reign of terror to the vast majority of peoples living throughout Europe and Scandinavia. The political, economic and religious forces of that time joined together to consolidate their power by eliminating those whom they perceived as impeding their ultimate objectives.

The unfortunate target of their efforts were the keepers of the healing arts and the ancient spiritual and cultural wisdom. Historians debate the exact toll of such a hellish time—whether it was several hundreds of thousands or as many as nine million—but what is undebatable is that the vast majority of victims were women. In fact, the Inquisition is now regarded as a period of genocide against women which successfully divested them of their power, self-respect, wealth, healing arts, prominence and influence in their communities.

The Inquisition guaranteed that the Church fathers were the undisputable spiritual authorities. It was also successful in enshrining medical knowledge securely in the realm of men since the Inquisition decreed that only trained medical doctors could now practice the healing arts. Needless to say, medical schools were barred to women (so, for that matter, was any formal education).

What a relief that such a violent and misogynist era ended long ago. Or did it? Unfortunately, it appears that some traditions linger on. Women of today are still prey to vast political and economic interests, suffering dire consequences to their health, financial independence and personal power. Perhaps the Inquisition hasn't ended at all, but merely taken a more subtle and devious form.

Certainly an astute observation was made by Sandra Coney in her book, *The Menopause Industry*, where she says, "the midlife woman is oblivious to the deeply sexist ideology underlying the options she has laid down before her. Naively she may think these are offered simply for her own benefit. She is not cognizant of the others who benefit or may also be served by her decisions. She is unaware, too, that the options themselves may be incompletely tested, that there may be considerable controversy about them in the medical literature and that doctors will differ in their views. What she is told—how much or how little—is mediated by her doctor. The end result is a woman poorly placed to decide for herself."

The influence of the medical and pharmaceutical interests exert on women is overwhelming. And it's no wonder. The fact is that women are very big business. The lucrative market spans all age groups of women from young teenagers to the postmenopausal. Synthetic hormones, surgical procedures, drugs, medical tests, diagnostic tests and on-going doctor's visits (not to mention the complications incurred from all of these) makes gynecology a most lucrative speciality.

Worldwide there are currently 400 million contraceptive users. Presently, 34.5 million American women are using some form of birth control.

Hysterectomies are another big industry. The Pill has been a significant contributor to conditions that later on necessitate the removal of a woman's uterus and ovaries. There are 22 million women in the United States whose have undergone hysterectomy, and 73 percent of women were also castrated (removal of ovaries) during the same surgery. Official statistics indicate that 620,000 women have surgeries for hysterectomy annually. However, that number does not include hysterectomies performed on an out patient basis. It's shocking to realize that presently one out of two women in the U.S. will have a hysterectomy by 60 years of age. What's even more shocking is that three quarters of the hysterectomies performed are on women under the age of 49. Removal of the uterus as well as the ovaries will immediately catapult a women into "surgical menopause" which necessitates hormones. What's more an oophorectomy (removal of the ovaries), medically classified as a castration, will also require more hormones.

Every day, approximately 6,000 women a day are reaching menopause.

The total cost from these chemical and surgical procedures is astronomical—billions upon billions of dollars. Gynecologists, hospitals and drug companies make more than $17 billion dollars a year from business of hysterectomy and castration. So it's no wonder that the medical industry views women as an unlimited resource to be plundered. When it comes to profits, unbiased controlled studies, long-term trials as well as natural alternatives are all sacrificed for the insatiable hunger for profits.

Nor is it an accident that gynecologists happen to be one of the highest earners of all specialists and that throughout a woman's life she is encouraged to be continuously medicalized. Natural female functions from menstruation through childbirth and then on into menopause are taken over by medical and pharmaceutical interventions. Barraged by a litany of false claims, emotive advertising campaigns, and, in some cases, downright lies, it's no wonder that so many women are thoroughly confused about matters relating to the health of their own bodies.

The History of Hormone Replacement

Perhaps there is no topic of greater confusion to women than the highly publicized introduction of Hormone Replacement Therapy for the menopausal woman. It has been receiving tremendous attention in our culture as the 'Baby Boomers' come of menopausal age. It is touted as the best thing for liberating women since the discovery of oral contraceptives (even though the statistics now show that wide use of the Pill has given rise to health hazards such as breast cancer, high blood pressure and cardiovascular disease on a scale previously unknown in medicine).[3]

Investigation into the theory of hormone replacement goes all the way back to the 1930's with the research of Dr. Serge Voronoff. His research involved implanting fresh monkeys testicles into men's scrotums with limited effectiveness. Offshoots of his research led to the grafting of monkey ovaries into women with rather dire consequences. After several fatalities (to both monkeys and women), the search was redirected to the use of synthetic estrogen. With the onset of World War II things were put on hold.

Menopause didn't really come into vogue as a topic of concern for the medical profession until the 1960's. In 1966 a New York gynecologist, Dr. Robert Wilson, wrote a best seller called *Feminine Forever*, extolling the virtues of estrogen replacement to save women from the "tragedy of menopause which often destroys her character as well as her health." Feeding upon women's greatest fears, his book sold over 100,000 copies the first year. Wilson energetically promoted menopause as a condition of 'living decay'. According to him, estrogen replacement was a kind of long sought after youth pill that would save poor fading women from the horrors of age. He popularized the erroneous belief that menopause was a deficiency disease.

Some of the menopausal myths which his book helped to enshrine amongst the general population as well as the medical community included:

❖ Ovaries shrivel up and die as a result of meno-pause.

❖ The woman becomes the equivalent of a eunuch.

❖ I have known cases where the resulting physical and mental anguish was so unbearable that the patient committed suicide.

❖ I have seen untreated women who had shriveled into caricatures of their former selves.

❖ Though the physical suffering from menopausal effects can be truly dreadful, what impressed me the most tragically is the destruction of the personality.

❖ To be desexed is to her a staggering catastrophe.

❖ She is incapable of rationally perceiving her own situation.

❖ The transformation within a few years of a formerly pleasant, energetic woman into a dull-minded but sharp-tongued caricature of her former self is one of the saddest of human spectacles.

❖ In a maze of longing and delusion they sometimes lose touch with reality and thus a menopausal neurosis develops.

Women's magazines eagerly seized upon his ideas and extensively promoted his concepts. This pleased Wilson immensely, having earlier set up the Wilson Foundation for the sole purpose of promoting the use of estrogen drugs. The pharmaceutical industry generously contributed over 1.3 million dollars to his foundation. Each year he received funds from companies such as Searle, Wyeth-Ayerst Laboratories and Upjohn which made hormone products that Wilson claimed were effective in treating and preventing menopause.[4]

Pharmaceutical companies jumped on the bandwagon with aggressive promotions and advertising campaigns. His message hit a receptive chord—mid-life women need hormone drugs to be rescued from the inevitable horrors and decrepitude of this terrible deficiency disease called menopause.

Wilson pioneered the use of 'unopposed estrogen' which is synthetic estrogen prescribed on its own. However, there had been no formal assessment of the safety of estrogen therapy or its long term effects. Unopposed estrogen went out of vogue when it became very apparent that it shortened the life-span of its users. In 1975, the *New England Journal of Medicine* examined the rates of endometrial cancer for estrogen consumers concluding that the risk was seven-and-a-half times greater for estrogen users. Women who had used estrogen for seven years or longer were 14 times more likely to develop cancer.[5] Wilson's theories then fell out of favor and the FDA told the drug companies that he was an "unacceptable investigator".

As the popularity of unopposed estrogen therapy waned, new approaches were sought. The focus was directed away from the false claims of preserving feminine beauty and youthfulness to relieving menopausal symptoms. The pharmaceutical industry resurrected Estrogen Replacement Therapy in the form of the new 'safe' Hormone Replacement Therapy, a combination of synthetic progesterone (progestin) and estrogen. HRT would supposedly protect menopausal women not only from cardiovascular disease but also the ravages of osteoporosis. The latest contentious discovery is estrogen's part in preventing Alzheimer's.

Another Perspective

While the so-called 'experts' on women's health are reassuring women that there are only very minor and insignificant side-effects, Dr. Lynette J. Dumble, Senior Research Fellow at the University of Melbourne in Australia, believes, "the sole basis of HRT is to create a commercial market that is highly profitable for the pharmaceutical companies and doctors. The supposed benefits of HRT are totally unproven." She believes that HRT not only exacerbates a woman's health problems but contributes to the acceleration of her aging process. HRT either hastens the onset of other medical conditions or worsens existing ones.

This perspective seems to be validated by the most recent findings from the National Institute of Health's sponsored *Boston Nurses Questionnaire Study* that followed 121,700 women for the past 18 years. The study revealed startling effects from HRT. It warned that women who used the combined progestin and estrogen of HRT increased their chances of developing breast cancer by up to 100 percent if taking the hormone for ten years or more. The study found ten years of use of estrogen alone increased the risk of breast cancer by 30-40 percent compared with women of the same age who never used postmenopausal HRT. Thus revealing that the combination of estrogen and progestin was risky business when it comes to breast cancer.

But even only five years of use has its dangers. The risk increased 30-40 percent if HRT is used five or more years. In women aged between 60-64 years the risk of breast cancer rose to 70 percent after five years of HRT. Finally, the study concluded that women using HRT were 45 percent more likely to die from breast cancer than those who chose not to use HRT or used it for less than five years.[6]

Dr. Graham Colditz, the study's principal researcher from Harvard recommends that women should only use HRT for relief of menopausal symptoms and for no longer than two or three years.

According to Leslie Kenton, the author of *Passage to Power*, "Everybody who is anybody will tell you that menopause is an estrogen deficiency disease and that you will need to take more estrogen as you approach mid-life. What may surprise you is this: not only is most of such commonly given advice on menopause wrong, a great deal of it can be positively dangerous."

Similar in his view of menopause is Dr. John Lee, retired physician and author of *What Doctors May Not Tell You About*

Menopause. "Menopause per se should be regarded as a normal adjustment reflecting a benign change in a woman's biological life away from child bearing and onward to a period of new personal power and fulfillment. The western perception of menopause as a threshold of undesirable symptoms and regressive illness due to estrogen deficiency is an error not supported by fact. More accurately, we should view our menopause problem as an abnormality brought about by industrialized cultures' deviation from a healthy lifestyle." The June 1996 *Townsend Letter for Doctors and Patients* points out that dietary, exercise and lifestyle factors have been shown to offer identical benefits to the proclaimed benefits of HRT without the risks.

It is becoming quite evident that there is another side to the Hormone Story—a perspective that can assist women of all ages to attain greater health and reclaim a greater sense of power, responsibility and dignity in their lives.

Chapter 2

A Brief Gynecological Tour of a Woman's Body

In order to understand the HRT debate and for that matter, the whole synthetic hormone issue, it is important to first have a rudimentary knowledge of a woman's body and its cyclic nature. As educated as we are as women, there seems to be a huge gap when it comes to having a meaningful and accurate understanding of the most intimate aspect of ourselves—our body.

Until recently doctors thought that menopause began when all the eggs in the ovaries had been used up. However, later work has shown that menopause is probably not triggered by the ovaries but by the brain. It seems that both puberty and menopause are brain-driven events.

So let us begin upon a fundamental understanding of the physiology of the female body.

The ovaries, located at either side of the uterus, are the primary sex organs. They are about 1 1/4 inches long and are shaped like prunes. At birth they contain all of the immature eggs, also known as follicles, that will mature and be released during a woman's fertile life. The developing fetus contains about seven million follicles; at birth the number of follicles are reduced to about two million. By the time puberty arrives there exists about 400,000 follicles, although only about 400 of them actually develop during a woman's fertile lifetime.

A follicle is a balloon-like sac which holds the immature egg in a protective fluid. As the egg follicles grow, they manufacture and release estrogen (estradiol) into the blood. After ten or twelve days, one of the developing egg cells out of the six to twenty that develop during a menstrual cycle moves to the outer surface of the ovary. The follicle then ejects the egg into the abdominal cavity where it finds its way into the fallopian tube for slow transportation to the uterus.

A normal menstrual cycle of every 26 to 28 days depends on a complex network of hormonal communications between the ovaries, the hypothalamus and the pituitary gland in the brain. All the hormones released are secreted not in a constant, steady way but at dramatically different rates during the 28 day menstrual cycle.

The development of the immature egg is initiated by the brain-controlled hypothalamus through a sex-gland-stimulating hormone called gonadotropin-releasing hormone (GrRH). GrRH then stimulates the pituitary to release two more substances into the blood stream. These two hormones are called follicle stimulating hormone (FSH) and luteinizing hormone (LH). Throughout the month, a constant feedback loop creates a continuous adjustment and regulation of the hormone levels between the brain and the ovaries.

On cue from FSH, estrogen triggers an egg to begin ripening, stimulates the buildup of tissue and blood in the uterus and controls the first part of the cycle. Estrogen production gradually builds to a peak just before ovulation then levels off for the remainder of the cycle, dropping again to low amounts at menstruation.

Estrogen also generates the changes that take place at puberty—the growth of breasts, the development of the reproductive system and the shape of a woman's body. Around the time of ovulation, estrogen also causes changes in the vaginal mucus, making it more tolerant of male penetration during sexual activity and more hospitable to sperm. As estrogen levels rise and ovulation is approached, the mucus becomes more profuse, thinner, wetter and clearer. At this time, just before ovulation and as estrogen peaks, the mucus becomes jellylike, resembling raw egg white, and can be stretched between the fingers. This is a signal that ovulation is imminent. This period of time from the beginning of menstruation until the onset of ovulation is called the follicular stage.

On the other hand, prompted by LH, the ovaries dramatically increase their output of progesterone at the time of ovulation about twelve to thirteen days into the cycle. Progesterone production during this phase of the cycle, called the luteal phase, leads to a refinement and 'ripening' of tissue and blood in the uterus. Progesterone also contributes to the changes in the vaginal mucus at the time of ovulation. The rise of progesterone at ovulation causes a rise in body temperature of about one degree Fahrenheit, a measure often used as one of the indications of ovulation.

Progesterone also plays a part in the mystery of the functioning of the follicles. Betty Kamen, Ph.D. author of *Hormone Replacement: Yes or No,* describes this process, "Follicles also communicate chemically with each other through a mechanism not yet fully understood. Only one follicle in one ovary continues to develop throughout the cycle. The egg-producing ovary sends a message to the other ovary to refrain from doing the same. The presence of progesterone initiates this "cease and desist" order. The growth of the chosen follicle continues to accelerate. During the last two days before ovulation, this follicle may be as large as three-quarters of an inch!"[1]

Immediately upon release of the egg on day fourteen, the fully matured follicle promoted by LH now functions in a different way. One of the wonders of the female body is the transformation of a follicle, upon release of the egg, into an endocrine gland called the corpus luteum which appears as a blister on the surface of the ovary. It is named corpus luteum because of its appearance as a small yellow, glandular mass. While it still continues to produce estrogen, it also becomes the prime production site of progesterone which dominates the second half of the menstrual cycle. When progesterone peaks, there is about 200 times as much progesterone as estrogen.

What is rarely understood is that the heightened sexual energy many women experience at the time of ovulation is the

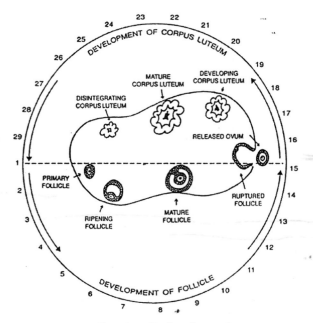

Ovarian Cycle - figure 1.

result of the surge of progesterone levels at the time of ovulation. Progesterone is the hormone necessary for increased libido, not estrogen as is commonly believed.

As the egg is ripening in the ovary, the uterus is ripening in preparation for the possibility of a growing fetus. The uterine lining thickens and becomes engorged with blood that will nourish a growing embryo. If no fertilized egg implants itself in the uterus, it then sheds its lining. This shedding is the blood of menstruation. Then the cycle begins again with the signal from the brain telling the ovary to begin ripening another egg.

According to Dr. Susan Love, author of *Dr. Susan Love's Hormone Book*, "It can take a while for this dance of hormones to get its choreography down. One study confirmed that earlier on girls have longer periods. The follicles don't mature and there may be a longer time between periods. This seems to be in part because the ovaries aren't yet really producing eggs and egg production is necessary for a regular "loop" to be completed. Once the whole system gets coordinated, a girl's cycles become regular and her symptoms settle down."[2]

If pregnancy occurs, progesterone production increases and the shedding of the lining of the uterus is prevented, thus preserving the developing embryo. As pregnancy progresses, progesterone production is taken over by the placenta and its secretion increases gradually to levels of 300 to 400 milligrams during the third trimester. It is also associated with the increased sense of well-being that women feel at this stage of their pregnancy.

As was previously mentioned, ovarian estrogen and progesterone stimulate the growth of the lining of the uterus in preparation for fertilization. Estrogen proliferates the growth of endometrium tissue and progesterone facilitates its further maturing so the fertilized egg can implant successfully. Adequate progesterone, therefore, is the hormone most essential to the survival of the fertilized egg and the fetus. It appears that the lack of adequate levels of progesterone at this time contributes to difficulties in conception and a high risk of miscarriage.

At around 40 years of age the interaction between hormones alters, eventually leading to menopause. It is still not clear how. Menopause may start with changes in the hypothalamus and the pituitary gland rather than the ovary. Scientists have conducted experiments where young mice have their ovaries replaced with those from aged animals that are no longer capable of reproducing.

The results showed that they were then able to mate and give birth. This shows that an old ovary placed in a young environment is capable of responding. On the other hand, when young ovaries were put into old mice, they were not able to reproduce.

Whatever the mechanism triggering menopause, as fewer egg follicles are stimulated, the amount of estrogen and progesterone being produced by the ovaries decline, although the other hormones continue to be produced. Estrogen levels drop to only 40-60 percent at menopause, just low enough so

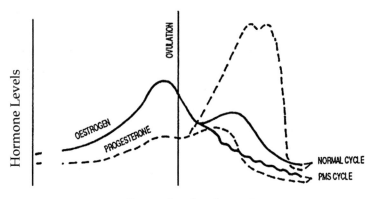

Days of cycle - figure 2.

that follicles do not mature, thus making pregnancy impossible. Contrary to popular belief, the ovaries do not shrivel up nor do they cease functioning. With the reduction of these hormones, menstruation becomes scantier and erratic and finally ceases.

Doctors who see the ovaries as useless after menopause point out that in women's older years the ovaries grow smaller. However, as women age, part of the ovary that shrinks is known as the theca, the outermost covering where the eggs grow and develop. The innermost part of the ovary, known as the inner stroma, actually becomes active at menopause for the first time in a woman's life. With exquisite timing, one function starts up as the other winds down.

After menopause the ovaries continue to function working in conjunction with other body sites such as the adrenal glands, skin, muscle, brain, pineal gland, hair follicles and body fat to produce hormones. Celso Ramon Garcia, M.D., Director of Surgery at the Hospital of the University of Pennsylvania, is one of the many authorities saying that the hormones produced by the postmenopausal ovaries promote bone health and skin suppleness, support sexual functioning, protect against heart disease and contribute to a woman's health and well-being.

The uterus is another misunderstood and denigrated organ by a medical profession which continues to reassure women that uteri are disposable organs that they can quite happily live without. Women are thus encouraged to embrace hysterectomies as a salvation to so many of their "female problems". *The People's Doctor Newsletter*, (Oct. 1989) report that what few women are aware of is that far from being a useless and unnecessary organ once a woman's childbearing days are over, the uterus is actually the main site for the production of the hormone prostacyclin which protects women from heart disease and unwanted blood-clotting. Since prostacyclin cannot be manufactured in a laboratory, the removal of the uterus will ensure its production will cease forever.

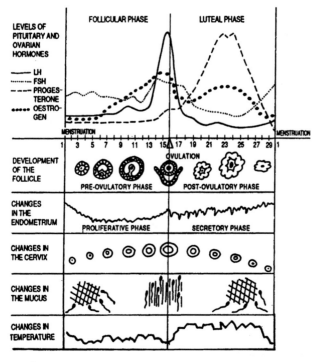

Female hormone levels during a monthly cycle - figure 3.

Provided a woman has taken good care of herself during the perimenopausal years with proper lifestyle, diet and mental and emotional health, the female body is quite capable of making healthy adjustments in hormonal balance after menopause.

Menopausal women have the opportunity to enter this phase of life empowered in their wisdom and creativity as never before. They have access to profound inner knowing.

The renowned sociologist, Margaret Mead, stated the now famous decree, "There is nothing more powerful than a menopausal woman with zest!" In many cultures around the world, menopause is a transition and an initiation into the fulfillment of a woman's power—totally symptom-free. She is held in the highest regard in her community as a wise, respected elder.

Unfortunately, as we will explore this natural adjustment of hormonal levels designed by nature to be a gradual and undramatic transition has been seriously altered for many women throughout the industrialized world.

Chapter 3

The Myth of Synthetic Estrogen and Progestins

The earlier research that led to the synthesis of estrogen made possible the development of the oral contraceptive in 1960. With the consent of the US Food and Drug Administration (FDA), the Pill was widely marketed as an effective, convenient method of birth control. True sexual liberation for women was at hand at last—or so we thought.

However, the entire basis for the FDA's consent was the result of clinical studies conducted on 132 Puerto Rican women who had taken the Pill for one year or longer. (However, there were five women who died during the study without any investigation into the cause of their deaths.)[1]

By the mid-1970's the death toll of women from heart attacks and strokes began to attract public notice. A newer, supposedly safer Pill was then created with a lower dose of estrogen. In fact, there has never been any valid scientific proof that the Pill was safe nor, for that matter, were any of the other forms of contraception presently available. Women are only now discovering the price they have been paying for their sexual freedom. By altering their hormonal balance, many varied and devastating emotional and physiological dysfunctions have been created.

It is 70 years since the first introduction of oral contraception and there are presently about 400 million women worldwide who are, in effect, 'trialing' the Pill. Its safety and long-term effects have still not been conclusively established.

It is interesting to note, however, that the Pill has produced a wide assortment of adverse effects and significant links have been established to breast cancer, high blood pressure and, in particular, cardiovascular disease, the major cause of female deaths.

Over 180,000 U.S. women are diagnosed with breast cancer every year and 46,000 deaths occur. Breast cancer incidence has gone up three percent a year every year since 1980. In 1940, a woman's life time risk of breast cancer was 1 in 16; that figure has now risen to 1 in 8.[1] Is this merely a coincidence or do these statistics indicate, perhaps, the harmful side effects of interfering with hormones?

While proclaimed as the primary missing ingredient for the menopausal woman, estrogen is also strongly recommended by the medical and pharmaceutical industries for the prevention of cardiovascular disease and osteoporosis. It is available in a variety of forms—pills, patches and implants. These days, most doctors will warn women of the inherent risks of going through menopause and, for that matter, the post-menopausal years without the essential protection of estrogen. Women are further reminded that menopause is a deficiency disease which supposedly means they are lacking estrogen and, therefore, must have supplemental doses to insure their health is maintained.

As Dr. Lynette Dumble has noted, "Broadly speaking, cardiovascular prevention in women has overwhelmingly focused on hormone replacement. Yet, as Elizabeth Barrett-Connor emphasizes, *The Big Trial*, the Coronary Drug Project of 1973 that included two estrogen regimens, was conducted on men. As part of *The Big Trial* design, estrogen doses extravagantly in excess of physiological levels were deliberately administered to men in order to induce gynecomastia (enlargement of male breasts) as an indication of successful feminization. This resulted in thrombosis and impotence and ultimately led to research failure because of treatment discontinuation amongst the study's participants."[2]

According to Dr. John Lee, the one notable study which formed the entire basis of the positive estrogen-cardiovascular link, known as the *Boston Nurses Questionnaire Study* and conducted with a large sampling of nurses, was radically flawed. Although there is ample evidence from numerous other studies showing that, indeed, the opposite is true—estrogen is a significant factor in creating heart disease—these findings have been virtually ignored in the frenzy for profits. He goes on to say that the pharmaceutical advertisements also neglected to mention the fact that stroke death incidence from that study was 50 percent higher among the estrogen users.

Dr. Lee has compiled a list of side-effects and physiological impairment which occurs from taking estrogen. These include increased risk of endometrial cancer, increased body fat, salt and fluid retention, depression and headaches, impaired blood sugar control (hypoglycemia), loss of zinc and retention of copper, reduced oxygen levels in all cells, thickened bile and gall bladder disease, increased likelihood of breast fibrocysts and uterine fibroids. Estrogen replacement interfered with thyroid activity, decreased sex drive, caused excessive blood clotting, reduced vascular tone and caused endometriosis, uterine cramping, infertility and restraint of osteoclast function.

With so many side-effects and dangerous complications, a woman must think very carefully about the HRT decision. Unfortunately, most doctors will say there is no other alternative and that it is relatively safe. While certainly most doctors are well meaning and sincerely concerned about their patients, their primary source of education and product information comes directly from the pharmaceutical companies. Since most women also lack essential education and understanding about their options, menopause can be perceived as a rather frightening and perilous time. Women fear that if they don't follow their doctor's advice (after all he really does know best), then they may face the remaining years of their life with the threat of great suffering and physical deterioration. Women are often in for a rude awakening when they experience firsthand just how badly their health needs have been managed.

Chapter 4

A Lesson From History

One of the greatest gifts of history is the ability to assess past events and past actions so that we can learn from our mistakes. The wisdom of hindsight can greatly assist us in making more appropriate choices to guide us safely into the future. Unfortunately, we rarely learn from the past and seem to be doomed to repeating our mistakes. When it comes to the widespread and indiscriminate use of synthetic hormones, there are many powerful lessons to draw upon.

One of the most poignant and tragic stories of synthetic hormones gone tragically wrong occurred with the introduction of a drug called diethylstilbestrol (DES for short), a synthetic estrogen prescribed to many pregnant women in the mistaken belief that it prevented miscarriage and pregnancy complications. The drug was widely prescribed for between four and six million pregnant women in the United States and Europe. Estimates in the US put DES exposure at between 2.7 and 5.4 percent of the total US population in 1979.

The DES story illustrates the failure of the medical profession, health authorities and drug companies to report the dangers, acknowledge the warnings and then take action to protect the public. This is also the story of a time-bomb still ticking away, not only in the innocent women who were administered the drug, but also in their daughters and sons with potential repercussions for generations to come.

Dishonest Beginnings

The story begins in the early 1940's, when Drs. George and Olive Smith, a husband and wife team from the Harvard Medical School, began theorizing about the use of a new drug, DES, in maintaining high-risk pregnancies. The maternity hospital associated with Harvard was used by the Smith's to test their theories.

Although DES was proved toxic in several early animal tests, these were largely ignored and DES was eventually marketed with the blessings of the FDA as a safe and effective drug to prevent miscarriage.

Dr. Robin Rowland, in her book, *Living Laboratories*, pointed out that "some of the women given this drug were used as experimental subjects and were told that they were taking a vitamin tablet." [1]

As the word spread throughout the medical community, DES was also prescribed as an estrogen replacement in menopause, as a 'morning after' pill (actually a five day treatment), to suppress lactation, as a treatment for acne, to treat certain types of breast and prostate cancer and to inhibit growth in young girls. It was primarily given in tablet form, but could also be injected or implanted. For several decades there was an additional use for DES. It was added to cattle feed as a 'growth promoter'.

The reason that DES has been likened to a time-bomb is that the drug companies assured the doctors that DES was perfectly safe. It has taken many years for the serious long-term effects of DES on the women themselves, as well as to their daughters and sons, to be revealed. And the story isn't over yet.

The Truth Comes to Light

In 1984, the first major study of breast cancer risks for DES mothers was published in the *New England Journal of Medicine*. It reported that some twenty years after taking DES, mothers had a 40 to 50 percent greater risk than non-exposed mothers. [2]

More shocking realizations about the indiscriminate use

of DES during pregnancy surfaced in the early 1970's. What had, up until then, been an exceptionally rare form of vaginal cancer occurring in women after menopause suddenly began appearing in young women (in all the world's prior medical literature there were only three cases reported developing in young women). Mysteriously, within a short period of time eight women were admitted to a Boston hospital diagnosed with this rare vaginal cancer. Their cancers were all traced back to the DES given to their mothers in pregnancy some 20 years earlier. Presently over 600 cases have been reported.

Since these initial ominous revelations, more effects of DES have emerged and been reported in medical journals. They include:[3]

1. Many DES daughters have benign tissue and structural damage to the vagina and cervix relating to their DES exposure.

2. Abnormalities of the uterus and fallopian tubes have been found, the common and characteristic change being a T-shaped uterus with a small uterine cavity. These abnormalities are suspected as possible causative factors in the higher incidence of pregnancy difficulties.

3. DES daughters, when compared with a non-exposed control group, experienced 3 to 5 times the rate of ectopic pregnancy; at least twice the rate of miscarriage in the first and second trimester; and at least three times the rate of pre-mature labor, premature birth or stillbirth. It appears that as many as 50 percent of DES daughters will experience these reproductive complications.

4. Recent research findings have revealed that DES daughters have between a two and fourfold increased incidence of squamous cell dysplasia and cervical cancer. This possibility was suggested

over a decade ago, following experiments with animals.

5. Approximately one third of DES sons have structural abnormalities of the genital tract including a history of undescended testicles (a known risk factor for contracting testicular cancer), cysts and lowered sperm counts. Some sons may be infertile.

6. DES exposure can also result in an impaired immune system. Certain conditions, including respiratory tract infections, asthma, arthritis and lupus were reported more frequently among the DES-exposed men and women.

What will happen to the DES daughters as they approach menopause? We won't have to wait too long before the answer becomes apparent.

At the 10th International Congress of Psychosomatic Obstetrics and Gynecology held in Stockholm in June 1992, various speakers gave the chilling news that to this day certain manufacturers of DES, unable to sell this drug in western nations for use in pregnancy, are successfully promoting and selling it throughout the third world! How much more human misery will the drug companies be responsible for?

All the warning signals are there. When it comes to the enthusiastic prescribing of synthetic hormones either in the form of estrogen, progestin or any others, are we doomed to repeat history as we once again interfere with women's natural hormonal production?

Chapter 5

Introducing Estrogen Dominance

The natural design of the body is to produce the two hormones, progesterone and estrogen, in a very sensitive and precise balance so that reproductive ability is maximized. These two hormones are closely interrelated in many ways and although they are generally antagonistic towards each other, each helps the other by making the cells of a target organ more sensitive.

Estrogen isn't really a single hormone. Estrogen refers to a class of hormones with estrus activity (i.e., proliferation of endometrial cells in preparation for pregnancy). These estrogens include estradiol and estrone, both of which are implicated in stimulating abnormal cell growth when found in higher than normal amounts in the body, and estriol which is known to be cancer inhibiting. Each type of estrogen has a different function in the body. These estrogens are produced mainly in the ovaries, although small quantities are secreted from the adrenal glands, the placenta during pregnancy and fat cells.

At puberty, estrogen in a girl encourages the development of breasts and the expansion of the uterus. Estrogen contributes to the moulding of female body contours and maturation of the skeleton. After that, estrogens help regulate the menstrual cycle and plays other necessary roles to maintain bone mass and keep blood cholesterol levels in check. When excessive quantities of estrogens, regardless of source, are present in a young woman's body they will contribute to the 'burn out' of her ovaries and undermine fertility.

In the case of progesterone, however, we are talking about one specific hormone. Thus, progesterone is both the name of the class and the single member of the class. In the ovaries, progesterone is the precursor of estrogen. Progesterone is also made in smaller amounts by the adrenal glands in both sexes and by the testes in males. It is also the precursor of testosterone and all important adrenocortical hormones. In addition to the sex hormones, corticosteroids are also derived from progesterone. Corticosteroids are essential for stress response, sugar and electrolyte balance and blood pressure, not to mention survival.[1]

While estrogen is the primary hormone during the first two weeks of a woman's menstrual cycle, fulfilling its role of preparing the endometrium for pregnancy, progesterone is the major female reproductive hormone during the latter two weeks of the menstrual cycle. Progesterone is necessary for the survival of the fertilized ovum, the resulting embryo and the fetus throughout gestation when production of the progesterone is taken over by the placenta.

One of the functions of estrogen is to store the energy derived from food as fat. This is why estrogen is readily given to cattle. Since cattle are sold by body weight, the more they're fattened up the more they're worth. Estrogen also adds weight by increasing water retention. It's no wonder estrogen has been so widely used in the meat industry (and a good reason to avoid all meat products that are not organically raised). Progesterone, on the other hand, turns fat into energy. Increasing progesterone levels contributes to weight loss and higher levels of energy.

There is a very delicate balance between the interplay of estrogen and progesterone. If that balance is interfered with, devastating effects occur. Unfortunately, introduced synthetic hormones, as well as environmental pollutants, are presently wreaking havoc with our hormones.

Growing Hormonal Imbalances

'Estrogen Dominance' is a term that was first used by Dr. John Lee. For the better part of the last two decades, Dr. Lee has been exploring the basis for the proliferation of such female problems as PMS, endometriosis, ovarian cysts, fibroids, breast cancer, infertility, osteoporosis and menopausal problems. From his clinical experience in the field of female health and from his published research, Dr. Lee believes that many women are suffering from the effects of too much estrogen. He finds that stress, nutritional deficiencies, estrogenic substances from our environment and taking synthetic estrogens combined with an ensuing deficiency of progesterone are the likely contributing factors to the creation of estrogen dominance.

Dr. Lee has discovered a consistent theme running through women's complaints about the distressing and often debilitating symptoms of PMS, perimenopause and menopause—too much estrogen, or estrogen dominance. Now, instead of estrogen playing its essential role within the well balanced symphony of steroid hormones in a woman's body, it has begun to over-shadow the other players, creating biochemical dissonance. The last thing a woman's body needs is more estrogen—either in the form of contraceptives or HRT. And when estrogen dominance symptoms appear, guess what is prescribed? Even more estrogen! The delicate natural estrogen/progesterone balance is radically altered due to this excess of estrogen. Progesterone deficiency is then exacerbated.

Some of the side-effects of unopposed estrogen include an influx of water and sodium into the cells, thus affecting aldosterone production, leading to water retention and hypertension. Estrogen causes intracellular hypoxia (oxygen deprivation), opposes the action of the thyroid, promotes histamine release, promotes blood clotting thus increasing the risk of strokes and embolisms. Estrogen unopposed by progesterone also decreases libido, increases the likelihood of breast fibrocysts, uterine fibroids, uterine (endometrial) cancer and breast cancer.[2]

Female Health Problems on the Rise

Female problems seem to be on the rise. Between 40 and 60 percent of all women in the western societies suffer from Premenstrual Syndrome (PMS). In addition, women can suffer from a whole plethora of symptoms—some menopausal and others not. Something quite alarming certainly seems to be happening to women. There are indications that the proper hormonal balance necessary for a woman's body to function healthily is being seriously interfered with by a number of factors.

When a healthy woman has her menstrual flow, it is the time of her cycle when she is making essentially very little, of either hormone. Estrogen production begins to increase about eight days after her period has started. Normally, from day 12 to day 26, there are hundreds of times more progesterone being produced than estrogen. So, if progesterone is missing, estrogen is then circulating continuously from day 8 to day 26. Essentially, if a woman has a whole month of nothing but estrogen, that woman will be estrogen dominant.

Research has revealed that a good portion of women in their 30's (some even younger)—long before menopause—will, on occasion, not ovulate during their menstrual cycle. Even though they still menstruate, they are not producing an egg. Without ovulation, no corpus luteum results and no progesterone is able to be made. This is called an anovulatory cycle. A progesterone deficiency will then ensue. The frequency of these anovulatory cycles increases as menopause approaches, changing the menstrual pattern to either a heavier or longer menstrual flow.

Several serious problems can result from anovulatory cycles. This will cause her to have menopausal symptoms such as weight gain, water retention and mood swings. It used to be true that the majority of women began menopause in their mid forties or early fifties. In the last generation, however, it appears that the pattern is changing. It is now becoming more frequent for women to be experiencing anovulatory periods in their early thirties without the cessation of periods (menopause) until their late fifties. Therefore, these women have a month-long presence of unopposed estrogen in their bodies with all the attendant side effects.

A progesterone deficiency can also seriously affect bones and is of great concern in the development of osteoporosis. Contemporary medicine is still largely unaware that progesterone stimulates osteoblast-mediated new bone formation. What that means is that progesterone actually stimulates the growth of new bone tissue and therefore osteoporosis can be reversed at any age. Lack of progesterone means that new osteoblasts are not created, potentially giving rise to osteoporosis.[3]

A third major problem results from the interrelationship between loss of progesterone and stress. When under stress, progesterone is converted into cortisol, the "fight or flight" hormone, at the expense of progesterone and estrogen. Stress combined with an unhealthy diet can induce anovulatory cycles. The consequent lack of progesterone interferes with the production of stress-combating hormones, thus exacerbating stressful conditions that give rise to further anovulatory cycles. Stress, nutritional deficiencies and chemical pollutants can all contribute to anovulatory cycles. And so the vicious cycle of progesterone deficiency continues.

It is important to note that, while the problem is recognized as a progesterone deficiency, it is not always true that progesterone levels are lower than normal but they may be low in comparison to elevated estrogen levels. Nevertheless, the delicate balance between estrogen and progesterone is significantly impaired. While not commonly understood by medical science, the growing incidence of anovulatory cycles, even in young women and the ensuing hormone imbalance is creating huge health problems. Women of all ages are now at higher risk of the entire range of estrogen dominant conditions. According to Dr. Lee, many of these common health problems can be offset by increasing the level of natural progesterone in the body.

Perimenopause

Menopause is not a sudden or unexpected event that occurs to a woman one day but rather a gradual process that may begin for her about ten years prior to the cessation of her periods, anywhere from the ages of thirty five through to her late forties. There are many factors that contribute to the hormonal changes occurring in her body. They include heredity, environment, lifestyle, the age at which she first menstruated, if she has given birth and if so, at what age and how many. Hormone levels are intimately connected to stress levels, nutrition and environmental toxins.

Dr. Jerilynn C. Prior, researcher and professor of endocrinology at the University of British Columbia in Vancouver, Canada believes that the distressing symptoms that women experience in the time leading up to menopause are in fact due to the presence of estrogen dominance in her body. Her pioneering work revealed that an alarming number of women from their mid-thirties onward are anovulatory. The significance of her findings is vital in order to understand the real cause of the many distressing symptoms plaguing women as well as the most effective ways to address the problem.

Dr. Lee's clinical observations, reinforce Dr. Prior's findings. "Anovulatory cycles occur when for whatever reason, a women does not ovulate, therefore, does not produce a corpus luteum from which progesterone is made. Progesterone levels then drop dramatically allowing estrogen to dominate the hormonal environment. Although she is usually still menstruating, an anovulatory woman may have irregular cycles or changes in her menstrual flow. During the many months of anovulatory periods, estrogen production may become erratic with surges of inappropriately high levels, alternating with irregular low levels. These anovulatory cycles contribute to the many symptoms of estrogen dominance which include breast swelling and tenderness, mood swings, fatigue, little or no desire for sex, headaches, sleep disturbances, water retention and a tendency to put on weight. In addition, estrogen dominance interferes with the thyroid action which increases her fatigue, makes her feel cold all the time and contributes to her weight gain. The most common age for the initial stages of breast and uterine cancer is five years or more before menopause, well before estrogen levels fall but coinciding with a drop in progesterone."[4]

The stressful lifestyle that has become the norm in society takes a terrible toll on women's health. Stress is a major contributor to major hormonal imbalances. Chronic exhaustion is epidemic as women struggle to maintain a career, family and marriage. Quiet, nurturing time with herself is more a fantasy than a reality. In an effort to maintain her lifestyle, her adrenal glands are constantly pumping out hormones that were meant to be used sparingly or for "flight or fight" situations. All to often this leads them to become tired, sluggish and depleted. Dr. Lee comments on this condition. "Her body gets the message that survival is at stake. Blood sugar becomes unstable. Digestion goes awry so she isn't absorbing nutrients properly. The ovaries respond by shutting down in favor of survival. When her ovaries shut down, progesterone production occurs only at the adrenals but they aren't working and she's not getting any progesterone from poor dietary habits, so she becomes progesterone deficient and estrogen dominant."[5] Bingeing on sugar, caffeine and refined carbohydrates further exacerbates the problem leading to an impaired metabolism.

Toxic estrogens, known as xeno-estrogens or estrogen mimics, presently found in large quantities in the environment add to the estrogen excess. These sources include pesticides, herbicides, auto pollution, polychlorinated biphenyls (PCBs) and nonylphenols found in many detergents. Exposure to these chemicals may result in enlarged ovaries, possible ovarian tumors, breast cancer and premature "burnout" of ovarian follicles, contributing to an early menopause. Males are not immune. Xeno-estrogens can contribute to atrophy of the testes, reduced sperm counts, small penises as well as cancer of the prostate and testes.

Anovulatory cycles also accelerate bone loss. Osteoporosis

is the consequence of low progesterone levels since it is the bone building hormone. In combination with poor diet and lack of exercise, many women arrive at menopause with osteoporosis well under way, already having lost 25-30 percent of their bone mass.[6]

Unfortunately many women are inappropriately diagnosed as having early menopause and thus prescribed HRT for their supposed "menopausal" symptoms. Taking more estrogen in addition to an already excess estrogen condition can not only lead to a worsening of the symptoms but can also contribute to more serious health problems. While hormonal problems are indeed widespread and a cause for concern, they are all too often symptoms of imbalance and poor health. Through reducing stress, improving diet and other lifestyle factors, using natural progesterone and receiving guidance from qualified practitioners of complimentary medicine, the perimenopausal woman can quite naturally, safely and effectively alleviate and even eliminate her symptoms.

Symptoms Caused or Made Worse by Estrogen Dominance

- ❖ Allergies
- ❖ Altered thyroid activity (mimicking hypothyroidism)
- ❖ Auto immune disorders such as lupus and thyroiditis
- ❖ Decreased sex drive
- ❖ Depression
- ❖ Dry Skin
- ❖ Endometriosis
- ❖ Excessive blood clotting
- ❖ Fatigue

- Fluid retention
- Foggy thinking
- Headaches
- Heavy or irregular menses
- Hirsutism (excessive hair growth on the body)
- Impaired blood sugar control (hypoglycemia)
- Increased body fat (especially around abdomen, hips and thighs)
- Increased likelihood of fibrocystic breast disease and breast tenderness
- Increased risk of endometrial cancer
- Infertility
- Loss of zinc and retention of copper
- Memory loss
- Miscarriage
- Osteoporosis
- PMS
- Premenopausal bone loss
- Reduced oxygen levels in all cells
- Reduced vascular tone
- Restraint of osteoclast function (ability to prevent the breakdown of bone tissue)
- Thickened bile and gall bladder disease
- Uterine fibroids
- Uterine cramping

Effects of Estrogen Dominance*

1. When estrogen is not balanced by progesterone, it can produce weight gain, headaches, bad temper, chronic fatigue and loss of interest in sex—all of which are part of the clinically recognized premenstrual syndrome.

2. Not only has it been well established that estrogen dominance encourages the development of breast cancer (thanks to estrogen's proliferative actions), it also stimulates breast tissue and can, in time, trigger fibrocystic breast disease—a condition which wanes when natural progesterone is introduced to balance the estrogen.

3. By definition, excess estrogen implies a progesterone deficiency. This, in turn, leads to a decrease in the rate of new bone formation in a woman's body by osteoblasts—the cells responsible for doing this job. Although most doctors are not yet aware of it, this is the prime cause of osteoporosis.

4. Estrogen dominance increases the risk of fibroids. One of the interesting facts about fibroids—often remarked on by doctors—is that regardless of size, fibroids commonly atrophy once menopause arrives and a woman's ovaries are no longer making estrogen. Doctors who commonly use progesterone with their patients have discovered that giving a woman natural progesterone will also cause fibroids to atrophy.

5. In estrogen-dominant menstruating women where progesterone is not rising and falling in a normal way each month, the shedding of the womb lining doesn't take place. Menstruation becomes irregular. This condition can usually be corrected by making lifestyle changes and using a natural progesterone product. Estrogen dominance is easily diagnosed by having a doctor

measure the level of progesterone through taking a saliva test.

6. Endometrial cancer (cancer of the womb) develops only where there is estrogen dominance or unopposed estrogen. This too can be prevented by the use of natural progesterone.

7. Waterlogging of the cells and an increase in intercellular sodium, which predisposes a woman to high blood pressure or hypertension, frequently occurs with estrogen dominance. This can also be a side effect of taking a synthetic progesterone. A natural progesterone cream usually clears up the problem.

8. The risk of stroke and heart disease is increased dramatically when a woman is estrogen dominant.

* Excerpt from *Passage to Power* by Leslie Kenton

Chapter 6

Adding Still Another Ingredient to the Hormone Soup

In addition to synthetic estrogens, women are now readily prescribed synthetic progestins, most commonly in the form of Provera. These progestins have been added to the estrogen formula to offset the hazards of estrogen drugs as previously mentioned. The pharmaceutical manufacturers themselves give a combined total of more than 120 potential risks and problems associated with HRT.[1]

At this point, it is important to make the distinction between the natural progesterone produced by the body and the synthetic progesterone-analogues classified as progestins, such as Provera, Duphaston, Primulut, Depo-Provera and Norplant. As you will learn, the two act differently in the body although doctors most often use the names 'progesterone' and 'progestin' interchangeably. Since natural progesterone is not a patentable product, the pharmaceutical companies have molecularly altered it to produce the synthetic progestins commonly used in contraceptives and HRT.

Synthetic progestins, because they are not exact replicas of the body's natural progesterone, unfortunately create a long list of side-effects, some of which can be quite severe. A partial list includes headaches, depression, fluid retention, increased risk of birth defects and early abortion, liver dysfunction, breast tenderness, breakthrough bleeding, acne, hirsutism (abnormal hair growth), insomnia, edema, weight changes, pulmonary embolism and premenstrual-like syndrome.

Most importantly, progestins lack the intrinsic physiological benefits of progesterone and cannot function in the major biosynthetic pathways as progesterone does. Progestins actually disrupt many fundamental processes in the body. Progesterone is an essential hormone that also plays a part in the development of healthy nerve cells, brain function and thyroid function. Progestins tend to block the body's ability to produce and utilize natural progesterone to maintain these life-promoting functions.

To appreciate the scope of the side-effects of progestins, it is instructive to review the entry for medroxyprogesterone acetate (Provera) in the Physicians' Desk Reference (PDR). An abbreviated list from the 1995 PDR follows:

Potential Side Effects of Medroxyprogesterone Acetate (Provera)

Warnings:

- Increased risk of birth defects such as heart and limb defects if taken during the first four months of pregnancy.

- Beagle dogs given this drug developed malignant mammary nodules.

- Discontinue this drug if there is sudden or partial loss of vision.

- This drug passes into breast milk, consequences unknown.

- May contribute to thrombophlebitis, pulmonary embolism and cerebral thrombosis.

Contraindications:

- Thrombophlebitis, thromboembolic disorders, cerebral apoplexy, liver dysfunction or disease, known or suspected malignancy of breast or genital organs, undiagnosed vaginal bleeding, missed abortion or known sensitivity.

Precautions:

- ❖ May cause fluid retention, epilepsy, migraine, asthma, cardiac or renal dysfunction.

- ❖ May cause breakthrough bleeding or menstrual irregularities.

- ❖ May contribute to depression.

- ❖ The effect of prolonged use of this drug on pituitary, ovarian, adrenal, hepatic and uterine function is unknown.

- ❖ May increase glucose tolerance; diabetic patients must be carefully monitored.

- ❖ May increase the thrombotic disorders associated with estrogen.

Adverse Reactions:

- ❖ May cause breast tenderness and galactorrhoea.

- ❖ May cause sensitivity reactions such as urticaria, pruritus, edema or rash.

- ❖ May cause acne, alopecia and hirsutism.

- ❖ Cervical erosions and changes in cervical secretions.

- ❖ Cholastic jaundice.

- ❖ Mental depression, pyrexia, nausea, insomnia or somnolence.

- ❖ Anaphylactic reactions and anaphylaxis (severe acute allergic reactions).

- ❖ Thrombophlebitis and pulmonary embolism.

- ❖ Breakthrough bleeding, spotting, amenorrhea or changes in menses.

When taken with estrogens, the following has been observed:

- ❖ Rise in blood pressure, headache, dizziness, nervousness, fatigue.

- ❖ Changes in sex drive, hirsutism and loss of scalp hair, decrease in T3 values (thyroid).

- ❖ Premenstrual-like syndrome, changes in appetite.

- ❖ Cystitis-like syndrome (urinary tact infections).

- ❖ Erythema multiform, erythema nodosum, hemorrhagic eruption, itching.

In an article entitled, 'Risks of Estrogen and Progestins' in the December 1990 issue of *Maturitas*, an English-language medical journal, several serious side-effects were mentioned. The author, Dr. Marc L'Hermite, found that 5 to 7 percent of women on conjugated equine estrogen (Premarin) could develop severe high blood pressure. When HRT was withdrawn, the women would return to normal readings.

An even more chilling study was reported in the May, 1996 *American Health Consultant Fax Bulletin*. A recent study involving rhesus monkeys indicated that contraceptives containing progestins (Depo-Provera and Norplant) could cause vaginal changes which may increase the risk of HIV infection in women. Fourteen of eighteen rhesus monkeys who had progestin implants caught simian immune deficiency (a close cousin to HIV) after the virus was administered into the vagina of the monkeys. The researchers stress that, while an animal model can provide useful information, the result is not immediately transferable to humans. However, U.S. Public health officials must not be telling the whole truth since they are now encouraging all women on contraceptives to use condoms as well. What is most interesting about this study is the obvious conclusion that due to the implants of progestins, the monkeys' immune systems were seriously compromised, thus making them susceptible to the virus. Since monkeys do not go through menopause they are never depleted of progesterone—except when their normal progesterone-building capacity and progesterone receptors are blocked—as occurred in this study. In the same way that synthetic progesterone impaired the normal hormonal functioning of the monkeys, synthetic progesterone as found in the form of human birth control blocks the body's production of its natural progesterone. Immune system impairment can be one of the disturbing side-effects.

While it is argued that estrogen has beneficial cardiovascular effects by increasing the good HDL cholesterol, when progestin is added this effect is reversed. Harmful lipoprotein changes resulting from progestins have been enough in some studies to actually increase heart disease risk.[2]

The *Boston Nurses Questionnaire Study* showed in its latest findings that adding progestin to estrogen not only failed to reduce women's incidence of breast cancer, but actually increased it. The study showed that 10 years of use of estrogen alone increased the risk of breast cancer by 30-40 percent while women who took estrogen and progestin increased their risk of breast cancer by up to 100 percent.[3]

According to Dr. Neil Lauersen, in his book, *"PMS, Premenstrual Syndrome and You,"* one of the problems with synthetic progestins is that they inhibit a woman's concentration of natural progesterone in the blood and, in fact, worsen the imbalance of female hormones and intensify the symptoms of PMS. Some progestins are actually 2,000 times more potent than progesterone, which is why certain progestins can make women feel more out of sorts."

Chapter 7

And The Synthetic Hormones Just Keep Coming

The medical profession's and pharmaceutical industry's love affair with women's hormones now adds another 'wonder' hormone to the growing list. The latest new recruit is testosterone—in the synthetic and most unnatural variety known as methyl-testosterone. It is either administered on its own or in conjunction with estrogen.

While women do manufacture testosterone in their bodies—from natural progesterone—it is only found in very small amounts. In come cases, such as hysterectomies or extreme hormonal depletion, a low dose natural testosterone may have a limited role. However, it is not without negative effects.

Dr. Lee makes the point that the fact that testosterone is now being included in hormone treatment, particularly for increasing bone density, as protection from cardiovascular disease and for treating fatigue, is an admission that estrogen by itself is not doing the job.

As is the case with all synthetic hormones, the side-effects of methyl-testosterone are quite alarming. Most of all, methyl-testosterone, which is administered either by injection or as a patch, is highly toxic to the liver, thus potentially causing serious liver damage or liver tumors. In addition, it can cause male pattern baldness, acne, excessive facial hair, enlarged clitoris and a permanent drop in voice pitch. There have been no conclusive studies showing the long-term safety of testosterone treatments.

Chapter 8

Hormone Addiction

Something which is little known about taking HRT is that it can be addictive. A former president of the London Royal College of Psychiatrists warns that estrogen used in HRT to counteract symptoms of menopause could be as addictive as heroin.[1]

In the 1970's testing was conducted on two groups of menopausal women. One group received estrogen replacement, the other group sugar pills (placebos). All were monitored for insomnia, nervousness, depression, dizziness, weakness, joint pain, palpitations, prickling sensations and hot flashes.

Both groups of women experienced an overall dramatic improvement during the first 90 days of the study, however the sugar pill group experienced more discomfort from hot flashes. When the groups were switched, those that had initially received estrogen experienced a pronounced return to their symptoms. It became apparent that once estrogen replacement stopped, a 'cold turkey' withdrawal effect was often experienced.

The same withdrawal effect has been found with implants, since the blood estradiol levels may become much higher than the body would normally produce.[2]

Nancy Beckham, herbalist, naturopath, homeopath and author of *Menopause: A Positive Approach Using Natural Therapies*, warns that, "Women on hormone replacement therapy who have enhanced well-being when their estradiol levels are very high but feel unwell when their blood levels are normal may be experiencing reactions similar to those of people on social drugs.

"It is well researched knowledge when you first have these drugs they give you a lift, which is pleasant; as you get used to the substance you find you need more to give you the same effect and ultimately your body craves a high level even though you may be unwell. When the substance in your blood drops below a certain level, you can experience withdrawal symptoms such as flashing, perspiration, sleep disturbance, shaking and other nervous reactions."[2]

While it is easy to prescribe HRT for women, there is hardly any medical data concerning the effects of stopping HRT in women who have received long-term treatment.[3] In one trial lasting three and a half years withdrawal lasted for six months.

Women must be advised to always taper off on their estrogen use and to never abruptly stop.

So, unknown to women, "menopause's little helper" could in fact be making estrogen junkies of them. It's great news for the pharmaceutical companies, but a calamity of untold proportion for women. Not only can they experience a wide range of physical symptoms, women may also suffer from psychiatric disturbances. Dr. Ellen Grant, author of *Sexual Chemistry*, was an early researcher of synthetic hormones and their effects on health. Dr. Grant has said, "when higher than expected rates of attempted suicide and violent deaths were recorded among HRT takers, the excuse was that more women suffering from depression are put on estrogens in attempt to treat them." Estrogens are rarely considered and therefore, overlooked as an extremely significant contributing factor in depressive behavior.

Chapter 9

Estrogen Dominance in the Environment

Another major factor contributing to an imbalance between estrogen and progesterone is environmental in nature. We, in the industrialized world, now live immersed in a rising sea of petrochemical derivatives. Petrochemicals are everywhere. They are in our air, food and water. Our machines run on petrochemicals, millions of products including plastics, microchips, medicines, clothing, foods, soaps, pesticides and even perfumes, are either made from petrochemicals or contain them. The popular slogan in the early 1950's, 'Better Living Through Chemistry,' is returning to haunt us.

These organochlorine chemicals include pesticides, herbicides (such as DDT, DDE, dieldrin, atrazine, methoxychlor, hetachlor, kepone etc.) as well as various plastics (polycarbonated plastics found in baby bottles and water jugs). These chemicals have an uncanny ability to mimic natural estrogen. As estrogen mimics, these compounds are highly fat soluble, non-biodegradable, accumulate in fat tissue of animals and humans and are difficult to excrete. They are given the name xeno-estrogens since, although they are foreign chemicals, they are taken up by the estrogen receptor sites in the body, seriously interfering with natural biochemical changes.

Mounting research is now revealing an alarming situation world wide created by the inundation of these hormone mimics. The best selling book, *Our Stolen Future*, written by Theo

Colburn of the World Wild Life Fund, Dianne Dumanoski of the Boston Globe and John Peterson Meyers, a zoologist, have identified 51 hormone mimics, each able to unleash a torrent of effects such as reduced sperm production, cell division and sculpting the developing brain.[1] Acting as endocrine disrupters, these chemicals interfere with hormones to upset growth, development, behaviors, intelligence and reproductive capabilities.

Disturbing Changes

Extremely disturbing events are being reported globally about other alarming changes happening in the environment.

In 1947, orthnithologists noticed that eagles in Florida had lost their drive to mate and nest. In the 1960's ranch minks that were fed fish from Lake Michigan failed to reproduce. In 1977, female gulls in California were nesting with females.

Not long ago, in Lake Apopka in Florida, wildlife biologists discovered that strange biological occurrences were happening to the alligators living there. In 1980, a toxic spill occurred dumping huge amounts of a pesticide similar to DDT into the lake. That event was almost forgotten until five years later when it was discovered that 90 percent of the alligators had disappeared. Most of those that remained were incapable of reproducing or had no urge to mate. The males were born with deformed penises that were 75 percent shorter than average. Further testing indicated that their testosterone levels were so low that they hormonally resembled females. Moreover, the females had abnormal ovaries and follicles described as "burned out."[2]

To add to this concern, recent reports show that strange hermaphroditic fish have been caught in Port Phillip Bay in Victoria, Australia. Similarly, a major British study revealed that male fish downstream from sewage treatment plants are changing sex as a result of estrogen chemicals which are not removed from treated effluent.[3]

Dr. Ana Soto, an endocrinologist at Tufts University, had

been experimenting with cancer cells taken from human breasts and then cultured. She found that they would grow when they were fed estrogens. As part of her experiment she quit feeding the cells estrogen. To her total amazement, however, the cancer cells continued to grow for four months even when no estrogens were fed to them. Dr. Soto then realized that the manufacturer of the flasks she had been using had started to use a different plastic—one that, when it becomes warm, releases minute quantities of the estrogen-like compound nonylphenol! Nonylphenols refer to a family of compounds that are used as surfactants (reducing the surface tension of water creating a bridge between two chemicals that don't normally mix) in pesticides as well as industrial and institutional cleaning products. Her tissues samples were being contaminated by the xeno-estrogens of the plastic flasks![4]

The Israeli Breast Cancer Finding

The first well-publicized study was conducted by two scientist, Jerome Westin and Elihu Richter at the Hebrew University School of Medicine. They were interested in the what they called the "Israeli breast cancer anomaly". During the late 1970's and early 1980's, Israel's breast cancer rate, particularly in young women, was much higher than that of other countries. They were perplexed by these alarming statistics.

The study showed that three organochlorine pesticides that produced over a dozen types of cancers in ten different strains of rats and mice were present in extraordinarily high concentrations in Israeli milk and dairy products. The three—benzene hexachloride, lindane and DDT—were present for 10 years in concentrations up to 100 times greater than in American diary products at the time. Concentrations in Israeli breast milk were possibly 800 times greater than in American breast milk. Embryos, fetuses and infants were particularly vulnerable to the carcinogens. One report indicated that organochlorine pesticides accumulated in the fetus to levels more than 100 percent higher than those found in the mother.

After a tremendous public outcry, the government was forced to ban the three organochlorines. The result was a precipitous drop in concentrations of these substances in cow's milk and breast milk of up to 98 percent.

Breast cancer rates also went down dramatically. Of 28 European and Middle Eastern countries surveyed, only Israel recorded a true decrease in rates between 1976 and 1986. Westin and Richter believed that the drop in breast cancer resulted from this decline.

Another observation was made from this study: all known factors contributing to breast cancer affect estrogen. The connection is stated by Greenpeace, "Exposure to hormonally active organochlorines early in life, especially in utero when hormonal feedback systems are being imprinted, can result in permanent alteration of systems that control estrogen and other sex hormones. Studies show increased risk of breast cancer among women born to mothers with indications of high estrogen levels during pregnancy. Thus, the transfer of accumulated organochlorines from mother to daughter may indeed contribute to breast cancer."[5]

The evidence is becoming indisputable. The legacy of this xeno-estrogenic pollution is permeating our very genes. There is an epidemic of reproductive abnormalities, including the steadily increasing number of breast, prostate, testicular and reproductive tract cancers, infertility, low sperm counts, poor sperm quality, the feminization of males and neurological disorders. The potential consequences of this overexposure are staggering, especially considering that one of the consequences is passing on reproductive abnormalities to offspring.[5]

What the Future Portends

Just how serious is this problem? In a May 1993 article in the British Medical Journal, *Lancet*, researchers in Scotland and Denmark hypothesized that xeno-estrogens are responsible for a steadily declining sperm count in men. According to Neils Skakkebaek of the University of Copenhagen, sperm counts have dropped by more than 50 percent since 1940. Meanwhile, the rate of testicular and prostate cancer in the United States and Europe has tripled in the past 50 years. Reproductive abnormalities such as undescended testicles have become increasingly common. Xeno-estrogens have also been implicated in impaired brain development in children.[6] They are also directly implicated in the 30 to 80 percent increase in breast, ovarian and uterine cancers in women over the past fifty years.[7]

In some rural communities in Australia, where heavy pesticide use has left residuals in drinking water, there have been reports of boys with abnormally small penises, along with the feminization of males and the masculinization of females.

A German study has shown that women with endometriosis have significantly higher levels of chemicals known as PCB's in their bodies. Seventy years ago, only 21 cases of endometriosis had been reported in the world. Now there are over 10 million cases in the US alone. Another group of xeno-estrogens called nonylphenols appear in spermicides, in diaphragm jellies, on condoms and in vaginal gels to facilitate dispersal.

This directly exposes the vagina and cervix to potent carcinogenic toxins.

A recent US Environment Protection Agency (EPA) data document revealed that US pesticide use reached an all-time high of 1,247 million pounds in 1995. This is over twice as much as was used 30 years ago when Rachel Carson's *Silent Spring* was published.[8] A study in the June 1996 edition of *Science* magazine showed that some combinations of hormone-distributing chemicals are much more powerful than any of the individual chemicals on their own. It revealed that combinations of two or three common pesticides, each at low levels which might be found in the environment, are up to 1,600 times as powerful together as any one individual pesticide by itself.

It is time for us to wake up and pay heed to these warnings for the sake of future generations. You can play your part in protecting your grandchildren and great-grand children in the same ways you can protect yourself by refusing to use pesticides, minimizing your use of plastics, purchasing hormone-free meat and organic produce, using "green" products for detergents and household cleaners and in general using 'natural' products in favor of petrochemical products.

Chapter 10

The Myth of Estrogen Deficiency

The trend these days is to strongly recommend hormone replacement therapy, featuring synthetic estrogens and progestins to all menopausal women. Unfortunately, this enthusiasm for drugs is not backed up by the facts. Estrogen deficiency is loudly proclaimed by medical practitioners, pharmaceutical advertising and many lay publications as the primary cause of all the symptoms attributed to menopause and post menopause—mood swings, depression, hot flashes, vaginal dryness, loss of sex drive and accelerating osteoporosis.

But is there really such a thing as estrogen deficiency? While it is true that menopause is associated with decreasing estrogen levels, it is not known whether these decreased levels of estrogen do in fact cause all the symptoms of menopause. Dr. Carolyn DeMarco, author of *Take Charge of Your Body* and a physician specializing in women's health issues, states, "there is no direct proof that estrogen lack causes heart disease or other ailments associated with the menopause."

Germaine Greer, writes that, "the proponents of HRT have never proved that there is an estrogen deficiency nor have they explained the mechanism by which the therapy of choice effected its miracles. They have taken the improper course of defining a disease from its therapy."

Dr. Jerilynn C. Prior points out that no study proving the relationship between estrogen deficiency and menopausal symptoms and related diseases has yet been done.

"Instead," says Dr. Prior, "a notion has been put forward that since estrogen levels go down, this is the most important change and explains all the things that may or may not be related to menopause. So estrogen treatment at this stage of our understanding is premature. This is a kind of backwards science. It leads to ridiculous ideas—like calling a headache an aspirin deficiency disease."[1]

Considering that western women tend to have a 10-15 year period prior to menopause when they are estrogen dominant and suffering from estrogen dominance symptoms, why are their doctors prescribing them still more estrogen?

During menopause, estrogen levels decrease to one-half to one-third of pre-menopausal baseline levels. While estrogen production falls only 40-60 percent, progesterone levels on the other hand, fall close to zero when ovulation no longer occurs.[2] Would it not be wiser to consider the progesterone loss effect when evaluating post menopausal symptoms and related conditions such as osteoporosis, heart disease, depression and loss of sex drive?

According to David Zava, Ph.D., director of research at ZRT Laboratory, who is developing saliva testing methods for monitoring levels of phytohormones in food and in the body, "It is interesting to note that Asian women have so few menopausal symptoms, despite the fact that their estrogen levels are, on average, only half the levels of Western women. "Hot flashes are not common in Asian countries. Pre and postmenopausal Asian women have only about half the circulating levels of estradiol and estrone (high levels are associated with an increased risk of breast cancer risk) in their bodies compared to American women. This might be the reason why they have a three to fivefold lower incidence of breast cancer.

"A recent paper by Lee-Jane Lu confirms that it is phytoestrogens in soy that are responsible for lowering estradiol levels. Soy phytoestrogens serve as a surrogate estrogen in their bodies and we think this is the reason they don't have cancer and they don't have heart disease and significant osteoporosis.

Asian women don't get endometrial cancer and men don't get prostate cancer."

The 'estrogen deficiency' hypothesis, as an explanation of most menopausal symptoms or health problems is, thus, not supported by the facts of estrogen blood levels by world wide ecological studies or by endocrinology experts. Has everyone jumped onto the 'estrogen deficiency' bandwagon without really understanding what is happening to women's hormones?

Chapter 11

But My Blood Tests Say...

Part of the confusion around HRT lies in the accepted way of measuring estrogen. Every woman who finds herself at the doctor's office suffering from menopausal symptoms will be given a blood serum test to determine her hormone levels. Serum is the clear, watery part of the blood without any of the red blood cells. When the ovaries make estrogen and progesterone for circulation in the watery blood serum, they bind them to protein to make them more water soluble. Protein-bound hormones are not biologically active; however, they represent over 90 percent of the hormones found in blood serum.[1]

What does all this mean? It means that, for the most part, blood tests to accurately measure the levels of hormones in a woman's body are useless and extremely unreliable. It is likely that your doctor may be unaware of this. The tests are only able to measure 1-9 percent of the biologically active hormones circulating in the body. Ninety percent or more remains undetected by these tests! So, most readings that may show low estrogen levels aren't measuring what's really there. Of course, the danger comes when a woman is prescribed hormones based upon test results which are erroneous. Even though her blood test may show low levels of estrogen, from which her doctor concludes she needs more estrogen (resulting in a prescription for estrogen), it is often the last thing in the world her body really needs.

"One prominent Californian gynecologist, skilled in

prescribing hormones, finally stopped trying to measure blood levels and began relying on a woman's description of the way she was feeling. She found this to be more accurate because blood levels varied so widely during a woman's cycle."[2]

Dr. Susan Love concurs. She says, "Blood tests for hormones are notoriously unreliable. Although (saliva testing) is a good way to measure them, I don't know why you would want to. There is no optimal estrogen level—only one which feels right for you. The dose of hormones you take should be balanced against your symptoms and not some arbitrary laboratory number determined by blood or saliva."[3]

So, how do you accurately test hormone levels? It is called 'saliva testing'. Hormones present in saliva reflect only the biologically available hormones. Saliva hormone tests are less expensive, very accurate and more relevant than serum tests for checking the accurate levels of hormones. It is able to confirm that any hormones being taken are being absorbed and utilized. Five years ago the World Health Organization began using saliva testing in place of blood serum testing.

If your doctor is unable to provide you with a saliva test, they can be ordered directly from the laboratories. You will then need to send your saliva test to the testing lab. The lab will check your saliva for hormone levels and send the results back to you. It is recommended that you discuss the confirmed results with your doctor.

Saliva tests and kits for both hormone and bone assays can be ordered from accredited laboratories. Trained health professionals will also be able to assist you in understanding the results and suggest appropriate treatment.

Blood Spot Testing

There is now a new type of blood spot test that accurately and more easily than ever, measures female and male hormone levels. It measures bioavailable hormones in capillary blood that is obtained with a nearly painless finger stick.

According to Dr. Zava, founder of ZRT Laboratory and

developer of the Blood Spot Test, "Unquestionably, saliva is an excellent means to assess the bioavailable fraction of hormones in the body, and our database clearly shows that salivary hormones are tightly linked with symptoms (e.g., low estradiol is associated with hot flashes, night sweats, vaginal dryness, bone loss, and sleep disturbances). However, in some cases, saliva may not be the appropriate body fluid to measure hormones, and some individuals are just unable to collect saliva due to dry mouth."

When it comes to accurately testing your hormones, there is now a choice. Some of you will want to continue using saliva to test your hormone levels, and others will prefer the blood spot test.

What's the Skinny on Bio-identical Hormones?

Beginning with the shocking results from the landmark Women's Health Initiative in 2002, the era of the modern miracle cure for menopause, Hormone Replacement Therapy, has continued to wane. A New England Journal of Medicine article (Feb. 2009) stated that the recorded drop in breast cancer rates was due to the reduction in the prescribing of HRT. According to the study's lead author, Dr. Rowan T. Chlebowski, long-term HRT probably caused breast cancer in 200,000 women between 1992 and 2002. It can be estimated that 44,000 women died during that decade due to taking synthetic HRT.

Another nail in the coffin for HRT was reported in the medical journal the Lancet. (Sept. 2009) by Dr. Apar Kishor Ganti, an Assistant Professor at the University of Nebraska Medical Center. Citing the latest study, which has found that women taking HRT who are diagnosed with lung cancer are more likely to die from that disease, Dr. Ganti states, "These results, along with the findings showing no protection against coronary heart disease, seriously question whether HRT has any role in medicine today."

So, if the nail is in the coffin of HRT, what about the popular alternative Bioidentical Hormone Replacement Therapy

(BHRT)? I am often asked this question. The key point to remember is that all estrogen replacement is now plant based-whether it is used in HRT or BHRT formulations. Estrogen is a powerful hormone. If, after assessing the results from either a saliva or blood spot hormone test, estrogen is determined to be low, then it might be appropriate to incorporate it as part of a treatment plan. But, it is always prudent to prescribe estrogen at the lowest possible dose for the shortest period of time!

Estrogen is estrogen is estrogen, so use it sparingly and only when absolutely necessary for the shortest amount of time is the safest way to receive the greatest benefit from this very potent hormone.

Chapter 12

The Pill—A Bitter Pill to Swallow

With hindsight, it will very likely be recorded in history that the widespread prescribing of synthetic hormones to women was the biggest medical bungle of the century. Most women taking oral contraceptives have very little idea about the hormones they are putting into their bodies, nor are they knowledgeable about the potentially serious side-effects.

A revolution was about to begin when the birth control pill arrived on the scene in 1960. It heralded an era that would emancipate fertile women from the burden of unwanted pregnancies thus opening the door to greater equality and freedom. For the past 40 years about 468 million women around the world have chosen the Pill as their preferred method of contraception. This "medical miracle" has enlisted almost 90 percent of Western women of reproductive age on some kind of contraceptive at some time in their lives.

The choices of the steroid hormone contraceptive has now expanded to include the combined and the low dose pill made with estrogen and synthetic progesterone called progestin or the mini pill either in the form of an implant or injection made only with progestins such as Depo-Provera or Norplant.

The Pill has been proclaimed as one of the most studied drugs in history. After three decades of experimentation (unfortunately on the unsuspecting pill users), we are told safe dosages are, at last, finally known. However, as the thin veneer of advertising hype, pharmaceutical cover-ups and sanitized clinical trials is peeled away, another picture emerges revealing the devastating consequences to women's health and well-being from the use of steroid hormones found in the Pill.

So, just what are the effects of suppressing natural hormones with synthetic ones? The Pill literally stops menstruation and bleeding only occurs each month because the synthetic hormones are not taken for seven days of the cycle. The bleeding that occurs would be more accurately termed 'withdrawal bleeding' not menstruation.

Taking the combined Pill increases the risk of coronary artery disease, breast cancer, cervical cancer, infertility, strokes, nutritional deficiencies and high blood pressure. The side-effects include nausea, vomiting, migraine-type headaches, breast tenderness, weight increases, changes in sex drive, depression, head hair loss, facial hair growth blood clots and increased incidence of vaginitis. Also, women with a history of epilepsy, migraine, asthma or heart disease may find that their symptoms worsen. Many of these effects may persist long after the discontinuation of the Pill.

According to Nancy Beckham, in her book *Menopause — A Positive Approach to Natural Therapies*, "Women on the Pill have a greater tendency to liver dysfunction and to more allergies. Estrogen drugs also affect vitamin concentrations. Vitamin A levels may be raised in the blood; vitamin B12 and C may be lowered. The clinical significance is not yet known." In addition essential fatty acids and zinc are depleted.

The introduction of Depo-Provera and Norplant, both of which are made from synthetic progestins, are equally disturbing to a woman's hormonal health, with all the previously listed side-effects and risks of progestins.

It is common practice today and has been for over a generation to prescribe birth control pills to women who complain of menstrual-related irregularities or discomfort. Under the prevailing misunderstanding about the real cause of women's problems, it is no wonder that this is the most accepted form of treatment. But, it's not really a treatment at all. It does not address the underlying imbalance—physiological and often emotional—which relates to estrogen dominance, poor diet and emotional stress.

It is important to recognize that the Pill is a potent artificial steroid drug which carries serious risks to a woman's health. Teenagers are especially vulnerable. The Pill is broken down in the liver which is consequently exposed to high doses of steroids. According to a report in the November 1995 *Natural Fertility Management* newsletter, the Pill causes 150 chemical changes in a girl's body. Many of these are not fully understood. The Pill seriously compromises a teenager's health, predisposing her to a lifetime of health problems. Teenager's need to be very fit and healthy to withstand all the metabolic changes in their bodies caused by the Pill.

The prevailing myth that the Pill is a safe and natural way to correct hormonal imbalances has lead to its widespread use in correcting teenager's menstrual cycles or alleviating painful periods. Puberty has now been medicalized. Even though nature often requires several years to help balance out a teenager's menstrual cycle, girls, as young as eleven years old, complaining of irregularities will all too often be recommended the Pill to supposedly help "regulate" their periods. Such common practices are both irresponsible and highly dangerous.

Since the breast tissue of young girls is still developing and is particularly sensitive to the over-stimulation from synthetic estrogen, the earlier a woman uses the Pill the greater the risk not only of developing breast cancer but also large tumors and a worse prognosis.

In a study by Olsson (*Cancer 1991*) it was shown that the Pill caused chromosomal aberrations in the breast tissue of young female users.

One study found the most terrifying results: the younger the women were at the time of diagnosis, the greater the possibility they would be dead within five years. John Wilks, author of "*A Consumer's Guide to the Pill and Other Drugs*" sums up this scandalous abuse of steroid hormones by stating that, "Given these results, it is not beyond the bounds of reasoned argument to suggest that this situation could be categorized as drug-induced vandalism of the female physiology. Yet little or nothing is heard of this lamentable betrayal of young women's health." Instead of relying upon the Pill to "regulate" problem periods, girls would be much better off to correct the problem at its source through improved diet, nutritional supplements, exercise and attending to emotional stresses. It would save them from the horrors of breast cancer and the high risk of dying from the disease.

A word is needed here about the trend that is occurring in our culture of early puberty in girls. According to Dr. Lee, "Early puberty results in longer lifetime exposure to estrogen produced by the ovaries, thus increasing cancer risk. It also appears that it leads to earlier follicle burnout and anovulatory cycles (menstruation without ovulation), starting as early as the mid thirties for most women. Just a generation or two ago, teenage girls didn't reach puberty until their late teens. Now they may start menstruating as early as 11 or 12. We have come to think of this as normal. It's not!

My suspicion is that this early onset of puberty is caused by exposure to the estrogens and xeno-estrogens so prevalent in every part of our environment from our meat supply (hormones are used throughout the meat industry in nearly all Western industrialized countries) to the air we breathe."

Francesca Naish, author of the book, *Natural Fertility*, reports that a 10-year program by the California Walnut Creek drug study of hospital admissions reports significantly increased inflammatory diseases in women under 40 who have taken or currently take the Pill. These inflammatory conditions include respiratory, digestive, urogenital and musculoskeletal disorders.

She goes on to say that, "The residue of the Pill can take three to six months to be eliminated from the system. This is the minimum amount of time that should lapse between coming off the Pill and conceiving, otherwise there are increased risks of fetal deformities.

"The Mini-Pill, which contains only progestins, is also often prescribed for lactating mothers and has been shown to severely deplete the nutrients available for the child in the mother's milk as well as providing the baby with an overdose of synthetic hormones. Synthetic progesterone is known to act on the hypothalamus, an important brain center and may masculinize a female infant and contribute to neo-natal jaundice."

We are only just beginning to realize the price we are paying for being part of a culture where fast food, fast cures and fast sex predominate. Certainly the long term effects of the Pill, in whatever form it comes, is still to be fully determined, not to mention the effects it may have on future generations. Is it worth the price that women must pay in terms of their physical, emotional and mental health for this form of contraception?

Most women will ask, "Well, just what are the natural alternatives to the Pill?" Barrier methods such as the diaphragm, cervical cap, condom and spermicide are certainly effective options. However, the most profound answer to that question requires a woman to gain a deeper understanding of the workings of her body and her natural cycles. It's learning about the various indications of fertile and non-fertile times. Owning one's fertility means to have an intimate relationship with one's own body. It requires taking responsibility for sexual intercourse. It also requires the ability to communicate with an understanding and receptive partner. It certainly is a totally different approach from the way most women address the issue of contraception and for that matter sexual relationships. It may require more effort but the benefits are immense.

If a woman's choice is to remain on the Pill, it is imperative that she take nutritional supplements that help address the pill-induced vitamin and mineral deficiencies. Health food stores carry formulas specifically for women who use the Pill. It is also recommended to come off the Pill after two years so that natural fertility cycles can be restored. It is also advised to seek consultation with qualified natural practitioners who can assess not only nutritional needs but also correct the functional imbalances. The Pill can interfere with the healthy functioning of the liver, pancreas, digestive system, ovaries, immunity and vascular systems.

If a woman is presently on the Pill and wishes to continue, it is extremely important to understand that the synthetic progestin in it will be taken up by all the progesterone receptor sites. Since progestins are synthetic analogues which means they are not exact matches of natural progesterone, they may interfere with the many bodily functions regulated by natural progesterone. It is no wonder that the Pill has such a long list of side-effects. Therefore, according to Dr. Lee, natural progesterone will have only limited or, in some cases, no benefit since the synthetic progestins have already and will continue to 'use up' the progesterone receptor sites.

There are, in fact, many natural birth control tools that offer a woman effective and safe contraceptive freedom. Natural fertility awareness programs and books teach the many indicators of fertile times. Through a combination of monitoring and charting temperature, mucus and even astrological influence of lunar cycles, a woman can be finely attuned to ovulation. During those fertile times, she can choose from a variety of barrier methods such as the condom, diaphragm, cervical cap or a spermicidal sponge.

In addition there are natural fertility techniques which incorporate various methods to naturally monitor fertile and non-fertile times rather than overriding or manipulating them. One of the best is Ovutech, a device the size of a lipstick tube that has a small microscopic lens at one end and a light at the other. If you are just about to become fertile or if you are fertile, you will easily see a beautiful crystalline ferning pattern under the microscope when applying saliva to the lens. This is an easy and convenient way to monitor hormonal changes and enhance awareness of your menstrual cycle. If you track your cycles and fertility on a calendar, there will be a keen awareness of where you are in your monthly cycle. Whether you are trying to conceive, avoid conception, or charting your cycles, the Ovutech is an inexpensive and reusable tool for fertility awareness. The ovutech should always be used in conjunction with charting temperature, cervical changes and mucus secretions.

Perhaps it is time for women to rethink the entire Pill issue. Two important questions worth asking are: "How precious is your health?" and "Are you willing to learn safe, natural forms of contraception?" The change that is needed to stop the exploitation of women's health for profits will require women as well as conscientious health professionals to make new, informed and safe choices. The health and well-being of millions of women around the world and the health of future generations depends on it.

Minor Side-Effects of the Pill

- ❖ Allergic reactions
- ❖ Breakthrough bleeding
- ❖ Decreased immune system function
- ❖ Disturbances in liver function
- ❖ Eye disorders such as double vision, swelling of optic nerve, contact lens intolerance and corneal inflammation
- ❖ Facial and body hair growth
- ❖ Fluid retention and bloating
- ❖ Fungal infections and tinea
- ❖ Hair loss
- ❖ Hayfever, asthma, skin rashes
- ❖ Loss of libido
- ❖ Lumpy or tender breasts
- ❖ Migraines
- ❖ Nausea
- ❖ Emotional disorders, depression, mood changes
- ❖ Secretions from the breast
- ❖ Skin discoloration
- ❖ Suicide is much more common among Pill-users than those using other forms of contraception

- Weight gain
- Systemic candida infection (candida or yeast infection)
- Urinary tract infection
- Venereal warts
- Vaginal discharges, including a much greater tendency to have vaginal thrush
- Varicose veins

Major Side-Effects of the Pill

- Disturbance to blood-sugar metabolism (possibly contributing to diabetes or hypoglycemia)
- Greatly increased chance of suffering a stroke (increasing with age and duration of Pill usage)
- Increased chance of hardening of the arteries and high blood pressure
- Increased risk of blood clots
- Increased risk of gall bladder disease (gall stones)
- Liver tumors (increasing with duration of Pill usage)
- Possible link with cancer of the endometrium, cervix, ovaries, liver and lungs
- Significantly increased risk of ectopic pregnancy
- Strong probability of more rapid development of pre-existing cancers and progression to cancer of abnormal cells
- Three-to-six fold increase in risk of heart attacks (according to age)
- Osteoporosis

Chapter 13

Enter Natural Progesterone

The present day prospects for a woman's health would indeed be gloomy if there were no other alternatives available. Fortunately, this is not the case. There exists a huge range of effective options. But to discover them, it is vital to look elsewhere than the traditional allopathic medical model. There is a long history of very successful treatments based upon a more natural approach to addressing the underlying symptoms. These include Naturopathy, Homeopathy, Traditional Chinese Medicine, Chiropractic, Herbalism and many more.

One of the most significant treatments presently available that safely and effectively addresses women's hormonal imbalances and related health problems is natural progesterone. In the early 1900's, research into the mysteries of women's hormones first revealed the existence of estrogen. Further investigations identified a second hormone which was proven to be necessary for a successful pregnancy, thus it was named progesterone (i.e. pro-gestation). Initial experiments extracted progesterone from sows' ovaries. It was then discovered that the placenta synthesized large amounts of progesterone. In the late 1930's, experimental work and clinical applications used progesterone obtained from the harvesting of placentas after childbirth and quick freezing them to extract the progesterone.

By 1939 it was discovered that an ingredient called diosgenin in the Mexican wild yam (Dioscorea villosa)—not to be confused with the average supermarket yam which is really a sweet potato—could be converted very easily and inexpensively into a molecule which is identical to the progesterone the body makes, now known as natural progesterone.

PMS is Real

The research and writings in the 1950's by pioneering British gynecologist, Dr. Katherina Dalton, first identified and coined the phrase 'Premenstrual Syndrome' (PMS). She was also the first to widely use progesterone with her patients. Dr. Dalton came to use progesterone through personal experience. She had noticed that her menstrual migraines disappeared during the last six months of her pregnancy when progesterone levels naturally soar. She first experimented on herself, discovering her migraines disappeared, and then found rapid and unequivocal effects when used with her women patients.

Thus began her decades-long and very vocal advocacy of this now international treatment. Since 1953, Dr. Dalton has become a leading investigator into PMS and a respected authority in the field. Besides establishing PMS as the most common of women's endocrine disorders, she was the first to show that PMS is the result of a progesterone deficiency and can be eliminated by increasing the levels of natural progesterone.

Progesterone Remembered

One present crusader committed to dispelling the erroneous beliefs about the cause and treatment of hormonal imbalance is Dr. John Lee. After 30 years of practice, Dr. Lee found that the women he saw through their child bearing years were now going through menopause and experiencing osteoporosis.

In 1982, after studying the work of biochemist, Ray Peat, Ph.D., on the importance of natural progesterone in bodily functions, Dr. Lee began using a transdermal natural progesterone cream derived from the wild yam to treat his osteoporotic patients.

He claims that, "After I had been in practice about 20 years,

I had more and more people who had osteoporosis. In 1976 and 1978, it became apparent to everybody in medicine that estrogen therapy, as we were instructed to give for osteoporosis, not only was not working very well for their bones but was the only known cause of cancer of the uterus. In my practice, I asked women who had osteoporosis to take the natural progesterone cream and I followed their bone mineral density tests just to see what would happen."

"It turned out that in three years time, the women typically gained 15 percent more bone. It wasn't just merely a delay of the osteoporosis, the bones actually became better. And in the process of following these women, I learned all the other things that progesterone did for them. They reported to me that fibrocystic breasts turned back to normal. Those that had acne or hair loss, male pattern baldness, showed me that their hair was coming back. These were things that at first I found unbelievable and yet when I researched them in our hospital library to find references to see if anyone had studied them, I found that, yes, they had been studied and, yes, they were known effects of progesterone."[1]

Dr. Lee, further states that along with increased bone density, these women were being relieved of their PMS, fibrocystic breast disease, hot flashes, vaginal dryness, depression, hypertension, migraines, hypothyroidism, high cholesterol and other menopausal symptoms.

Dr. Lee became even more convinced of the efficacy of natural progesterone when he found that many women could decrease their estrogen and finally discontinue it entirely and still maintain their bone density. Though estrogen is often deemed necessary for vaginal dryness and hot flashes, he also saw these problems improved with just the use of natural progesterone.

Dr. Lee conducted independent research into the many applications of natural progesterone. His non-pharmaceutically funded research presents a much broader understanding of a woman's hormonal options and offers a totally safe, effective alternative that is free of all side effects. Together with a good diet and some lifestyle changes, he has found that this natural hormone is capable of eliminating much of the suffering associated with both PMS and menopause.

A Recurring Theme

Dr. Lee's research led him to the realization that there was a consistent theme running through women's complaints of the distressing and often debilitating symptoms of PMS, perimenopause and menopause—the presence of too much estrogen in the body (estrogen dominance). He was convinced that, instead of estrogen playing its essential role within the well balanced symphony of steroid hormones, it overshadowed the other players, creating biochemical dissonance. Adding more estrogen to a woman's body, either in the form of contraceptives or HRT, was the last thing she needed.

However, the prevailing myth of estrogen deficiency means that when estrogen dominant symptoms appear, such as hot flashes, menstrual difficulties, depression etc., guess what is prescribed? More estrogen! The delicate natural estrogen/progesterone balance is radically altered due to too much estrogen. Progesterone deficiency is then exacerbated.

For many years, Dr. Lee has been sounding the alarm, with little support and much resistance from his medical colleagues.

However, while the erroneous focus has been on estrogen, natural progesterone seems to have been totally overlooked by medical science. Considering that natural progesterone is non-patentable and inexpensive, it is not surprising that this is so. It is important, however, to have a much greater understanding of and appreciation for this remarkable hormone.

It is also important to remember that it is progesterone that is responsible for maintaining the secretory endometrium which is necessary for the survival of the embryo as well as the developing fetus throughout gestation. It is little realized, however, that progesterone is the mother of all hormones. Progesterone is the important precursor in the biosynthesis of adrenal corticosteroids (hormones that protect against stress) and of all sex hormones (testosterone and estrogen). This means that progesterone has the capacity to be turned into other hormones further down the biochemical pathways as and when the body needs them. The point needs to be emphasized that estrogen and testosterone are end metabolic products made from progesterone. Without adequate progesterone, estrogen and testosterone will not be sufficiently available to the body. Besides being a precursor to sex hormones, progesterone also provides many other important intrinsic physiological functions.

Supplementation with natural progesterone corrects the real problem—progesterone deficiency. It is not known to have any side-effects nor have any toxic levels been found to date. Natural progesterone increases libido, protects against fibrocystic breast disease, helps protect against breast and uterine cancer, maintains the lining of the uterus, hydrates and oxygenates the skin, reverses facial hair growth and thinning of the hair, acts as a natural diuretic, helps to eliminate depression and increases a sense of well-being, encourages fat burning and the use of stored energy, normalizes blood clotting and is a precursor to other important stress and sex hormones. Even the two most prevalent menopausal symptoms, hot flashes and vaginal dryness, quickly disappear with applications of natural progesterone.

Thus progesterone has many diverse and beneficial actions throughout the body. Since progesterone protects against the undesirable side effects of unopposed estrogen, whether produced by the body before menopause or as a consequence of estrogen supplementation or xeno-estrogens from the environment, it will assist the body to return to greater hormonal balance. All of the undesirable effects of estrogen are countered by progesterone. Restoring proper progesterone levels is restoring hormonal balance.

Functions of Progesterone

❖ is a precursor of the other sex hormones, including estrogen and testosterone

❖ maintains secretory endometrium
(uterine lining)

❖ is necessary for the survival of the embryo and fetus throughout gestation

❖ protects against fibrocystic breast disease

❖ is a natural diuretic

❖ helps use fat for energy

❖ functions as a natural antidepressant

❖ helps thyroid hormone action

❖ normalizes blood clotting

❖ restores sex drive

❖ helps normalize blood sugar levels

❖ normalizes zinc and copper levels

❖ restores proper cell oxygen levels

❖ protects against endometrial cancer

❖ helps protect against breast cancer

❖ assists to builds bone and is protective against osteoporosis

❖ is a precursor of cortisone synthesis
(in the adrenal cortex)

❖ reverses hirsutism (excessive hair growth)

Chapter 14

Discovering Some of the
Benefits of Natural Progesterone

Clinical research and personal experience are presenting more and more convincing evidence about the multiple roles natural progesterone plays in the body. Many important discoveries about progesterone's place in creating and maintaining health have been forgotten along the way, overshadowed by estrogen's starring role.

One of the problems with medicine is that it tends to label hormones by their presumed functions, thus there is the tendency to classify hormones either as sex hormones or thyroid hormones, etc. However, the body is a more complex and interrelated organism—hormones do so many things. For instance, brain cells concentrate progesterone and testosterone to levels 20 times higher than the blood carries. Imagine, progesterone receptors in the brain! Obviously brain cells wouldn't do this unless progesterone and testosterone has some important job to do there. This latest research helps to unravel the curious findings from many of Dr. Lee's patients who reported increased concentration, mental alertness and other improved mental abilities while using progesterone! Perhaps the foggy thinking so often associated with menopause is merely another sign of progesterone deficiency.

Growing interest is stimulating the enthusiasm for more research. It might even be said that at long last progesterone is coming of age! Without a doubt, more information about progesterone's role in creating health will be revealed in the years ahead. The following are some of the known benefits natural progesterone provides.

Aches and Pains of the Muscles (Fibromyalgia)

When stretching any distance, nerve cells are sheathed in an off-white insulating covering called myelin which protects the nerves from trauma and chemical erosion as well as preventing short-circuiting of the electric impulses along the way. Along the nerves throughout the body are special cells called Schwann cells which continually maintain the myelin sheath. Progesterone receptors are on the Schwann cells, allowing them to perform their function.

It is no surprise, then, to discover that fibromyalgia, inflammation of the nerve cells in the muscle accompanied by aches and pains, is the result of a progesterone deficiency. The traditional medical approach uses non-steroid anti-inflammatory drugs, anti-depressants and a variety of stress management techniques without great success. Dr. Lee found that fibromyalgia, which is reaching epidemic proportions in the United States, would disappear within six months to a year upon using progesterone supplements.

Allergies

Allergies are produced in the body when the allergen (the allergy-producing substance) load exceeds the capacity of the body to deal with it. Adequate cortisone blocks the histamine response to allergens. Progesterone is a precursor not only to estrogen and testosterone, but also to all the corticosteroids made by the adrenal glands. Adrenal exhaustion is the result of stress, vitamin C deficiency and progesterone deficiency. Progesterone assists in alleviating allergy problems.

Arthritis

Arthritis is a condition of aching joints or an ache of the connective tissue around the joints. Doctors usually prescribe non-steroid anti-inflammatory drugs. The origins of such symptoms have a variety of causes. One such cause is the lack of physiological (made by the body) cortisone responses to check the inflammatory reactions. Natural progesterone has anti-inflammatory properties that the synthetic analogues do not have. In addition to his own experience, Dr. Lee, has had many doctors report that women have experienced significant relief from aches and pains.

Auto Immune Disorders

Auto immune disorders occur when one's own antibodies attack the organs and tissues in the body. Auto immune disorders are generally found more often in women. The onset of such disorders, such as Lupus, Graves' Disease, Hashimoto's thyroiditis or Sjorgren's disease are more prevalent in middle age and are related to estrogen supplementation or estrogen dominance. Recent studies have shown that women who use hormone replacement therapy are more likely to get lupus.[1]

Hormone researcher, Dr. Ray Peat, professor of biochemistry at Blake College in Oregon has found, "The thymus gland is the main regulator of the immune system. Estrogen causes it to shrink while progesterone protects it."[2]

Candida

A common problem for many women these days is a condition called candida. It is the proliferation of yeast growth due to several factors. Vaginal cells contain glucose which is a favorite nutrient of candida. Estrogen dominance increases mucus glucose levels, encouraging candida growth. When hormonal imbalance is restored to normal balance using progesterone, candida growth is less likely to persist.

Endometriosis

A serious condition in which tiny islets of endometrium (the inner lining of the uterus) become scattered in areas where they don't belong—the fallopian tubes, within uterine musculature and on the outer surface of the uterus and other pelvic organs, the colon, the bladder and the sides of the pelvic cavity.

With each monthly cycle, these islets of endometrium respond to ovarian hormones exactly as endometrial cells do within the uterus—they increase in size, swell with blood and bleed into the surrounding tissue at menstruation. The bleeding (no matter how minor) into the surrounding tissue causes inflammation and is very painful. Symptoms begin 7 to 12 days before menstruation and become excruciatingly painful during menstruation.

Sometimes doctors will recommend the radical decision of a hysterectomy for severe cases of endometriosis.

All other options should be fully explored first. A hysterectomy is a major trauma for a woman's body. Dr. Lee has had considerable success treating endometriosis with natural progesterone. "Since we know that estrogen initiates endometrial cell proliferation and the formation of blood vessel accumulation in the endometrium, the aim of the treatment is to block this monthly estrogen stimulus to the aberrant endometrial islets. Progesterone stops further proliferation of endometrial cells."

Dr. Lee advises women to use natural progesterone cream from day six of the cycle to day 26 each month, using one ounce of cream per week for three weeks, stopping just before their period begins. This treatment requires patience. Over time (four to six months), however, the monthly pain gradually subsides as monthly bleeding in these islets lessens and healing of the inflammation occurs.[3]

It is interesting to note that endometriosis is cured by menopause due to reduced estrogen levels.

As previously mentioned, there is also a connection between increased xeno-estrogens, particularly nonylphenols, dioxins and endometriosis. Considering that endometriosis is a twentieth century disease, it is obvious that environmental factors should be seriously considered.

Christiane Northrup, M.D., author of *Women's Bodies, Women's Wisdom*, considers endometriosis an illness of competition.

She believes that "it comes about when a woman's emotional needs are competing with her functioning in the outside world. When a woman feels that her innermost emotional needs are in direct conflict with what the world is demanding of her, endometriosis is one of the ways in which her body tries to draw her attention to the problem. A great many of the women I've seen who have endometriosis drive themselves relentlessly in the outer world, rarely resting, rarely tuning in to their innermost needs and deepest desires."[4]

Fibroids

Fibroids are round, firm, benign (non-cancerous) lumps on the uterine wall, composed of smooth muscle and connective tissue. They are rarely found singularly. While they are usually small in size, they can grow to the size of a grapefruit. They often cause, or are coincidental with, heavier periods, irregular bleeding and/or painful periods. More than 40 percent of women over the age of fifty have these benign growths. They are also the most common reason for performing a hysterectomy and usually the most unwarranted reason.

Dr. Lee states that fibroid tumors are, "Another example of estrogen dominance secondary to anovulatory cycles and consequent progesterone deficiency. They generally occur 8 to 10 years before menopause."[5]

Natural progesterone offers a better alternative. Fibroids are a product of estrogen dominance, which is why they disappear after menopause. However, if estrogen is supplied after menopause, fibroid tumors will be stimulated to grow. When sufficient natural progesterone is replaced, fibroid tumors no longer grow in size and often will shrink. Natural progesterone used in conjunction with dietary changes which includes a high fiber, no fried foods, primarily vegetarian and organic diet is quite effective in reducing fibroids. Other natural remedies which include Western herbs, nutritional support, homeopathic remedies and Chinese herbs have also provided successful treatment.

Hair Loss and Increased Facial Hair

Through lack of ovulation (anovulatory cycles) progesterone levels fall. The decrease in progesterone signals the adrenals to increase the production of an androgen (male-like) hormone called androstenedione. This adrenal cortical steroid produces male characteristics such as male pattern hair loss and increased facial hairs especially the dark ones appearing on the chin. When progesterone levels are raised through the use of natural progesterone, the adrenal hormone production will gradually fall. Although it usually takes four to six months to restore normal hair growth patterns, head hair will grow and facial hair will disappear. Increased androstenedione levels at menopause contribute to the thinning of hair and increase facial hairs of postmenopausal women. Along with an improved diet and proper nutrition, natural progesterone cream will help reverse this condition.

High Blood Pressure

Estrogen dominance is one of the many causes of high blood pressure or hypertension. Estrogens and progestins adversely affect cell membranes. Milton Crane has extensively studied the effects of estrogen, progestins and progesterone on cell membranes and high blood pressure. He has concluded that estrogen dominance and oral contraceptives are a major cause of hypertension in women.[6]

If you are on diuretics or other anti-hypertensive drugs and using progesterone, it is wise to have your doctor monitor your blood pressure, so as to reduce or eliminate your anti-hypertensive drugs gradually as appropriate to prevent low blood pressure.

Estrogen dominance or synthetic progestins substituting for progesterone impair the functioning of cell membranes, causing increased levels of sodium and water in the cells. This results in intracellular edema, a build up of fluids in the cells leading to hypertension. Dr. Lee estimates that 90 percent of all cases of essential hypertension are probably due to unrecognized hormonal imbalance.

Hot Flashes

Hot flashes are one of the most prevalent symptoms of hormonal change in western culture. It is interesting to note that Japanese women do not experience hot flashes and, in fact, have no word for it. As menopause is approached and even 5 to 10 years afterwards, it is estimated that around 80 percent of western women experience this sudden rise of heat in the body, with up to 40 percent suffering sufficiently to seek assistance from a health professional.

The hot flash is still not totally understood. Diminished estrogen levels play a role. Withdrawal of estrogen causes an increase in the levels of the hormones FSH and LH. The brain center that regulates the secretion of these hormones, the hypothalamus, directs many body functions including body temperature, sleep patterns, metabolic rate, mood and reaction to stress. The higher the levels of FSH and LH, the more blood vessels dilate or enlarge, raising body temperature, which increases blood flow to the skin—the hot flash.

The part of the hypothalamus involved in these hormonal changes monitors progesterone as well as estrogen. Since the post menopausal woman continues to make estrogen in respectable levels and makes little or no progesterone, hot flashes may respond well to progesterone supplementation alone. Hot flashes will also respond to much smaller levels of supplemental estrogen when progesterone is added.

Not all hot flashes are related to decreases in estrogen levels. Hypothyroidism can be a cause, as can alcohol intake and out-of-control diabetes. In fact, waves of heat may hit anyone, of any age, who engages in behavior that forces the temperature-regulating system to step up its activities.

The most common triggers for hot flashes include spicy foods, caffeine, chocolate, alcohol, drugs of all kinds, hot drinks, hot weather and stress. Irregular eating can also desta-bilize your blood sugar, causing hot flashes. One of the biggest culprits is sugar. Sometimes just regulating sugar intake is enough to successfully control hot flashes.

Some of the other natural ways to alleviate severity and frequency of hot flashes include three to four hours of exercise per week, deep breathing and a healthy diet which includes plenty of fresh vegetables and fruits. Extensive research has also shown vitamin E—contained in whole grains, nuts and seeds, sweet potatoes and crab meat—can reduce hot flashes.

Stress is a major trigger in upsetting the balance in the body. Stress factors, such as busy schedules, emotional upsets and lack of adequate sleep and relaxation, all contribute to hot flashes. For a woman, looking after her emotional as well as physical needs is of paramount importance.

Infertility, Early Miscarriages and Post Natal Depression

All the above conditions relate to low progesterone levels. According to Dr. Lee, "Estrogen dominance caused, once again, from progesterone deficiency has resulted in a near epidemic of infertility among women in their mid thirties. Excess estrogen seems to stimulate the ovaries to over-produce follicles, which, combined with delayed child bearing, results in an early burn out of follicles.

"I had a number of patients who had been unable to conceive. For two to four months I had them use natural progesterone from days 5 to 26 in the cycle (stopping on day 26 to bring on menstruation). Using the progesterone prior to ovulation effectively suppressed ovulation. After a few months of this, I had them stop progesterone use. If you still have follicles left, they seem to respond to a few months of suppression with enthusiasm and the successful maturation and release of an egg occurs. Some of my patients who had been trying to conceive for years had very good luck with this method. There are even few children named after me!"[7]

The chief cause of early loss of pregnancy is now thought to be luteal phase failure in which ovarian production of progesterone fails to increase sufficiently during the first several weeks after fertilization. Maintaining the secretory endometrium (uterine lining) and the development of the embryo are dependent upon adequate luteal-supplied progesterone. The failure of progesterone production during this critical time of pregnancy mirrors the rising incidence of progesterone deficiency occurring ten or more years before menopause. Other contributing factors are stress, nutritional deficiencies and xenoestrogens.

When several miscarriages have occurred, Dr. Lee recommends progesterone supplementation (in addition to nutritional support), starting after ovulation (day 14 or so) and continued on after pregnancy is confirmed for an additional two months. After two months, placenta-driven progesterone becomes dominant. Reducing the supplemental progesterone during the third month should be gradual so as to avoid any abrupt drop in progesterone levels.[8]

As pregnancy advances, placental production of progesterone rises to a level of 350 to 400 milligrams a day (normally 20 milligrams) and the ovaries' contribution at that point is nil.

After delivery, the placenta-derived progesterone is suddenly gone. Since the adrenals are the primary source of progesterone at that time, if they are exhausted there would be insufficient progesterone produced. Remember that progesterone is a natural anti-depressant.

Many women experience depression in the days and weeks following childbirth. Research by Brian Harris and his colleagues in Wales found that, among 120 women, those with the highest prenatal and lowest postnatal progesterone levels also scored highest on measures of postpartum depression scores.[9]

Post partum depression is generally difficult to treat and often antidepressants become the first line of defense. Natural progesterone would be a more sensible and safer approach.

Migraine Headaches

When migraine headaches occur with regularity in women only at premenstrual times, they are most likely due to estrogen dominance. Estrogen causes dilation of the blood vessels and thus contributes to the cause or causes of migraines. One of the many beneficial qualities of natural progesterone is that it helps restore vascular tone, counteracting the blood vessel dilation that causes headaches. Natural progesterone is certainly a more natural way to treat these migraines and avoids the need for more dangerous pharmaceutical drugs.

Ovarian Cysts

Ovarian cysts are products of failed or disordered ovulation. They may be asymptomatic or create pelvic pain. Some may grow to the size of a golf ball. Such cysts occur when, for reasons presently unknown, the ovulation did not proceed to completion.

To understand this cystic condition, it is essential to have an in-depth appreciation for the hormonal process. Each month one or more ovarian follicles are developed by the effects of follicle-stimulating hormone (FSH). Another hormone, luteinizing hormone (LH), is responsible for promoting ovulation and the transformation of the follicle (after ovulation) into the corpus luteum, the progesterone-producing structure. With each month's surge of LH, the follicular site swells and stretches the surface membrane, causing pain and possible bleeding at the site of the cyst.

The signalling mechanism that shuts off ovulation in one ovary each cycle is the production of progesterone in the other. If sufficient natural progesterone is supplemented prior to ovulation, LH levels are inhibited and both ovaries think the other one has ovulated, so regular ovulation does not occur.

Adding natural progesterone from day 10 to day 26 of the cycle suppresses LH and its luteinizing effects. Thus, the ovarian cyst will not be stimulated and, usually within a month or two, will regress and atrophy without further treatment.

Premenstrual Syndrome

PMS is identified by a collection of symptoms that usually occur one week to ten days before the menses. The most common symptoms include several or all of the following: bloating, weight gain, headache, backaches, irritability, depression, breast swelling or tenderness, loss of libido and fatigue. The full range of symptoms include confusion and disorientation, poor judgement and decision-making, mood swings, body aches, anger and verbal abuse, lethargy alternating with increased energy, alienation, guilt (at having abused friends), lack of self-esteem and cravings for sweets, especially chocolate. Further, every system in the body can be affected: immune, digestive, circulatory, nervous, endocrine and dermatologic (skin). Women experiencing PMS may experience any combination of the above and with varying degrees of severity, from mild to overwhelming.[11]

What is interesting to note about these symptoms is that they are the same as symptoms of estrogen dominance.

In his practice, Dr. Lee would measure the weight gain of his patients in the luteal phase of their cycle (the two weeks before the onset of menstruation). If he found that there was an increase in weight of three to six pounds at that time, he would conclude that the patient had PMS. The weight gain was the result of intracellular fluid retention (the swelling of all the cells in the body). The swelling of brain cells can result in the commonly reported PMS feelings of anger, irritability and hostility. Sound familiar? Natural progesterone also helps to alleviate these symptoms.

PMS is certainly an indication that there is significant hormonal imbalance occurring in the body.

Natural progesterone has proven to be highly effective when included in a regime for restoring hormonal balance. "In my practice, hundreds of women who were severely handicapped by PMS have been completely symptom-free with natural progesterone," reports Neils Lauersen, M.D., professor of obstetrics and gynecology at the New York Medical College. In his practice more than 90 percent of his patients who have tried natural progesterone have found relief.

Joel T. Hargraves, M.D., director of PMS and Menopause Clinics at Vanderbuilt University in Nashville, Tennessee, has also found impressive results using natural progesterone. "I've been using natural progesterone for 12 years and I haven't seen any long-term effects. It doesn't affect cholesterol levels, it doesn't affect Mother Nature—basically it is a wonderful thing."

A leading proponent of natural progesterone, Dr. Katarina Dalton has found that, "target cells containing progesterone receptors are widespread in the body, although most are found in the brain, particularly in the limbic area which is the area of emotion, rage and violence. The other receptor sites where progesterone should be received are the eyes, nose, throat, lungs, breast, liver, adrenals, uterus and vagina. All these are areas in which symptoms of PMS may occur such as headaches, asthma, laryngitis, pharyngitis, rhinitis, sinusitis, mastitis, alcohol intolerance and congestive dysmenorrhoea."[12]

While it is likely that a hormone imbalance directly or indirectly caused by progesterone deficiency is the major factor in the majority of PMS cases, there may also be other factors that deserve attention, especially in those cases that do not find complete relief with progesterone treatment. Contributing factors to PMS include poor nutrition as well as physical and emotional stress.

Sex Drive (Low Libido)

Sex drive or libido, although mediated by sex hormones, is really a brain function. The underlying primary sexual drive in all mammals emanates from the brain centers mediated by sex hormones. The effect of progesterone on human libido has been largely ignored by mainstream medical research. The accepted belief is that estrogen is the primary sex drive hormone in women.

What is rarely understood is that the heightened sexual

energy many women experience at the time of ovulation is the result of the surge of progesterone levels at the time of ovulation. Progesterone is the hormone necessary for increased libido, not estrogen as is commonly believed.

In studies with hamsters which had their ovaries removed, estrogen alone was insufficient to restore sexual receptivity; progesterone was required.[9] Dr. Lee reports that his patients' flagging libido returned only when progesterone was added. While testosterone is usually given the spot light as the key hormone for turning on libido, the role of progesterone is overlooked (remember that progesterone is the precursor of testosterone).

Skin Problems

When acne appears in women in their late thirties or forties, increased androgen (masculinizing hormone) is suspect. Dr. Lee has found that in almost all his female patients with this condition, supplemental progesterone cleared the skin. His hypothesis is that ovarian follicle depletion, leading to progesterone deficiency, results in increased adrenal production of androgens. When progesterone is resupplied, androgen production goes down and the skin clears.

Seborrhea is a condition that causes flaking and itching skin without specific inflammation of the skin follicles. It, too, clears rapidly with topical progesterone cream.

Used as a skin cream, natural progesterone has a wonderful moisturizing effect on the skin. It increases hydration and oxygenation of the cells. Women using the cream have been impressed with the improved appearance of their skin. They have reported to me that wrinkles are disappearing! Natural progesterone has been an ingredient in moisturizing creams for the past 45 years.

Thyroid Deficiency

Thyroid is the hormone that regulates metabolic rate. Low thyroid tends to cause low energy levels, depression, cold intolerance and weight gain. In his medical practice, Dr. Lee noticed that there were greater numbers of women taking thyroid supplements for hypothyroidism than men. He also recognized that many estrogen dominance symptoms, such as fat and water retention, breast swelling, headaches and low libido were present. When progesterone levels were increased, not only did their estrogen dominance symptoms decrease or disappear but so too did their presumed hypothyroidism.

Estrogen, progesterone and thyroid hormones are inter-related. Estrogen causes food calories to be stored as fat while thyroid hormone causes fat calories to be turned into usable energy. Thyroid hormone and estrogen have opposing actions. Dr. Lee has hypothesized that estrogen inhibits thyroid action in the cells creating hypothyroid symptoms despite normal serum levels of thyroid hormone. Symptoms of hypothyroid-ism occurring in his patients with unopposed estrogen (pro-gesterone deficiency) lessened when progesterone was added and hormone balance was restored.[13]

Vaginitis, Vaginal Dryness and Thinning

There is a higher incidence of vaginitis in women taking the Pill, which often relates to the Pill's suppression of natural hormones. After menopause, women are more predisposed to vaginal dryness as well as vaginal, urethral and urinary tract infections, although these are not inevitable consequences of menopause. Dr. Lee has noticed that, "Those who opted for natural progesterone therapy have been remarkably free of these problems. Further, their previous vaginal dryness and mucosal atrophy return to normal conditions after 3-4 months of progesterone use. Progesterone cream can also be used effectively and safely intravaginally. This suggests that natural progesterone also provides a direct benefit to vaginal and urethral tissues or may sensitize tissue receptors to the lowered levels of estrogens still present in post menopausal women."[14]

In addition, a diet rich in whole grains and vegetables is

essential. Also, you can topically apply aloe vera gel or insert a vitamin E soft-gel capsule vaginally. (The PH of your body will break down the capsule so there is no need to puncture it) or use a vitamin E suppository.

Maca, a well known Peruvian herb, has adapagenic properties that restores endocrine balance and repairs the vaginal tissue.

Dr. Earl Surwit a professor at the University of Arizona's College of Medicine specializing in pelvic floor disorders and incontinence conducted a clinical study investigating alternatives to vaginal estrogen creams. He found that a natural vaginal ointment called MoisturePom (made by Pomegranate Health), a pomegranate lipid complex made from extracts of pomegranate fruit and pomegranate seed oil successfully restored vaginal lubrication and promoted healthy vaginal tissue. It also had a positive effect on incontinence and helped to strengthen pelvic floor muscles. Dr. Surwit found that in every way, MoisturePom was as effective as estrogen creams without raising estrogen levels.

If none of the recommended natural solutions are effective, then you can request a prescription for estriol cream which is applied internally. A 1991 Norwegian review concluded that estriol is a safe, cheap and effective therapy for the symptoms of estrogen deficiency after menopause including atrophy of the vagina, urethra and bladder, urinary tract infections and abnormal function of the lower urinary tract. The researchers found that estriol had no metabolic effect or serious side effects at recommended doses and was safe for use long term.[15]

Chapter 15

Suggested Uses of Natural Progesterone

Natural progesterone, as stated earlier, is synthesized from the Mexican wild yam or soy. The most effective way to use natural progesterone products is absorption via the skin. Absorption through the skin is 40-70 percent more effective than ingestion. This is because the liver removes a high percentage of ingested hormones, returning them to the digestive tract where they are converted to water soluble forms that bind with other substances and are then eliminated from the body.

The most popular and effective progesterone products are available as creams, oils or roll-on's. In dermal transport, progesterone is first absorbed into the subcutaneous fat layer and then passively diffused throughout the body via the blood circulation. With continued use, fat levels of progesterone reach an equilibrium and successive doses of progesterone result in increased blood levels and stronger physiological effects. This is why progesterone applications may require two or three months of use before maximum benefits are experienced.

Every woman's body is unique. It is important for her to find the right dose for her body. The suggested dosages are merely guidelines. Women who are experiencing more severe symptoms may initially require larger or more frequent amounts. It is considered safe to experiment until the dose that is correct for your body is determined. It may also be necessary to try different products until the most desired results are experienced.

How to Apply it?

Natural progesterone is most readily and easily absorbed by the thinner skinned areas of the body where there are plenty of capillaries. These include the areas where we tend to blush. The best areas are the face, neck, chest, abdomen and the upper and inner areas of the arm and thighs. Creams can be used as excellent moisturizers for the face. It is best to rotate the sites, applying cream to one area one day and another area the next day, etc.

When to Use it?

Application of natural progesterone follows the body's natural progesterone production. Since menstruation is the time of lowest levels of progesterone, it is advised that it not be used during this time. Application begins upon cessation of menstruation, which is usually day 8 of the menstrual cycle. Smaller amounts are applied two times daily for the next two weeks. During the last week of the menstrual cycle (day 21 to 28), the amount is increased, again following the body's own natural progesterone cycle. Depending on the concentration of progesterone in the product, 1/8 to 1/2 teaspoon is used per day, or 3 to 10 drops of oil. Roll-on application suggests an 8 inch strip once or twice daily. Be sure to follow the instructions that are provided with the product you are using.

If a woman no longer has periods, she can either follow the calendar month or count the day she begins as day one and apply natural progesterone for the next three weeks. It is advised to have one week off. However, some menopausal women find that they need to use the product daily in order to alleviate symptoms.

Hormone Replacement Therapy — How to Get Off It

Hormone Replacement Therapy is a combination of an estrogen and a progestin such as Provera. If a woman is taking both estrogen and a progestin, the first step is to substitute natural progesterone for the progestin, then gradually decrease the estrogen. Dr. Lee advises his patients to reduce the estrogen they are taking by 50 percent and to immediately stop using the progestin at the time they begin using natural progesterone. He has found no ill effects in stopping the progestin abruptly.

Then the next month they can reduce the estrogen again by 50 percent and the same for the next. By the end of the third month, the HRT can be safely and completely discontinued. Continue using the natural progesterone. It is recommended to use a 2 ounce jar a month over the three months. The cream can be applied for 21 days twice daily with a break of 7 days which will ensure that the hormone receptors are sufficiently stimulated. When a woman has successfully weaned herself off the HRT, she may then find that her body requires less cream.

When a woman on HRT wishes to stop taking it, there are a few things that need to be kept in mind. The first thing is that the progestins and natural progesterone compete for receptor sites in the body, so the full benefits of progesterone will be reduced until the progestins have been cleared from the body.

Secondly, blood levels of natural progesterone will not rise to optimum levels until 2 or 3 months after you begin to use the cream.

Thirdly, the use of natural progesterone cream may temporarily sensitize the estrogen receptors, leading to an experience of high estrogen effects—fluid retention, tenderness and swelling of the breasts, or even the appearance of scant vaginal bleeding. These are only temporary and will normally soon clear.

If a woman has had a hysterectomy and prescribed only an estrogen replacement, she can follow the same protocol as for weaning off of HRT, adding the natural progesterone and reducing her estrogen by half each month.

It is important to allow time for the levels of natural progesterone to reach physiological equilibrium as the synthetic hormones are reduced. Generally if the estrogen is stopped abruptly (and no natural progesterone is added) women will tend to experience symptoms of rapidly falling estrogen levels such as hot flashes, migraines and vaginal dryness. These symptoms are a form of withdrawal. It is not recommended to go 'cold turkey'.

If after three or four months, the natural progesterone does not eliminate all the symptoms, then Dr. Lee suggests that a woman may consider adding a little estrogen, usually in the form of estriol (the safest form of estrogen). However, most women report that the natural progesterone alone success-fully addressed all their symptoms and were feeling better than ever.

Hysterectomies

Hysterectomies are the most common major non-obstetrical surgical procedure in the United States, second only to cae-sarean section. About 20 million American women have had their uteri removed. Officially about 750,000 hysterectomies are performed annually. Unofficially, however, the figure is closer to one million. The average age at which women have this operation is 42. More than three-quarters of hysterectomies are performed on women under the age of 49. In fact, twice as many women in their 20's and 30's are hysterectomized as women in their 50's and 60's. It is estimated that fifty percent of American women will have a hysterectomy in their lifetime.

Dr. Stanley West, noted infertility specialist, Chief Of Reproductive Endocrinology at St. Vincent's Hospital, New York and author of The *Hysterectomy Hoax*, says, "more than 90 percent are unnecessary." He believes that, in general, a hysterectomy is never necessary unless a woman has cancer. Other more conservative views conclude that 50 to 90 per-cent should not have been done. According to John Robbins in his best selling book *Reclaiming Our Health*, "What all the authorities agree upon is that 90 percent of the procedures are elective, that there are alternatives in at least 90 percent of the cases, and that less than 10 percent of the operations are, in fact, medically imperative."

Technically, a hysterectomy is the removal of the uterus

and an oophorectomy or ovariectomy is the removal of the ovaries. Removal of the ovaries is also known in medical terminology as female castration. However, popular parlance now refers to the removal of the uterus and ovaries as a "total hysterectomy." Since women who have hysterectomies go into instant, surgically induced menopause, they are immediately put on estrogen replacement therapy (ERT) although estrogen (or any other drug or other treatments) will never successfully replace a woman's ovarian and uterine hormones or functions. Since estrogen has been implicated in endometrial cancer, only women without a uterus are now prescribed estrogen on its own without a progestin although estrogen still puts women at increased risk of breast cancer. Estrogen will also cause many women to experience all the ensuing estrogen dominant symptoms.

In whatever form it may occur, a hysterectomy is radical surgery for a woman. Women experience a loss of physical sexual sensation as a result. The procedure also tends to shorten, scar and dislocate a woman's vagina.

Some of the most common consequences, in addition to operative injuries are: heart disease, osteoporosis, bone, joint and muscle pain, painful intercourse, displacement of bladder, bowel and other pelvic organs, urinary tract infections, chronic constipation and digestive disorders, short term memory loss, depression and dulling of emotions.

The leading reasons for recommending hysterectomies are fibroids (usually the cause of heavy bleeding), endometriosis, and uterine prolapse (the uterus falls from its normal position). Fibroids and endometriosis respond extremely well to natural progesterone cream as well as dietary and other nutritional support. A prolapsed uterus, in addition to following dietary and nutritional guidelines, has been successfully treated with naturopathy, Traditional Chinese Medicine and other natural healing modalities. Obviously, a woman has a right to be informed of these effective and much less invasive alternative treatments.

Usually women with hysterectomies are told by their

doctors that they must remain on estrogen for the rest of their lives. However, this is not true. Dr. Lee has his patients wean themselves off the synthetic hormones by gradually reducing the dosage (following the same protocol as described for coming off HRT). In those very few women who still have hot flashes or vaginal dryness, he gives them some estrogen cream, usually estriol to use intravaginally for a few months. They are then able to taper off the estriol completely. Natural progesterone combined with a good diet, exercise, appropriate nutritional support and stress management will insure women who have had hysterectomies as well as oophorectomies renewed hormonal balance without ever needing synthetic hormones.

Menopause

All women experience menopause differently. Some women's bodies require higher progesterone levels than others. The correct amount for one woman is not necessarily the right amount for another. The cream can be applied according to the calendar month and applied over a 14 to 21 day time period. Then discontinue application until the next month.

For vaginal dryness or discomfort, the cream can be applied intravaginally. This may be in addition to or instead of your daily applications.

If hot flashes or night sweats are severe, women have found relief by applying the cream every fifteen minutes for the next hour following the episode.

Some women find that they require increased amounts of cream daily to find relief from their symptoms. These women may need to use the cream for the entire month rather than taking 7 days off.

When progesterone levels are increased, estrogen receptors become more sensitive—that is, they are more likely to respond to estrogen. Thus, some women notice that after a week or two of applying progesterone, some vaginal bleeding may occur due to their own estrogen levels. At that point, a woman may stop the progesterone for a week or two and then start again for a three week period.

During the week while being off of the progesterone, there may be some bleeding. This is due to the persistence of estrogen production, which will diminish over time. This is the advantage of stopping progesterone for one week each month. It allows the estrogen-induced blood buildup to be shed.

In cases of persistent spotting or vaginal bleeding (for more than three months), consult your physician.

Osteoporosis

Three of the best methods to accurately determine the degree of bone loss in osteoporosis are serial dual photon absorptiometry (DPA), dual energy x-ray absorptiometry (DEXA) and ultrasound densitometry. These tests measure bone density very precisely, are relatively low in cost and emit minimal radiation. It is suggested that, if possible, you have one of these tests done before you begin using the cream in order to establish a base line from which to measure changes in bone density. Subsequent tests may be performed at six month or one year intervals so you and your physician can monitor bone growth, however, testing is not mandatory to begin using the cream.

For people with mild osteoporosis or for prevention of osteoporosis, follow the general recommendations for the natural progesterone. If you have severe osteoporosis or have experienced fractures, the daily amounts can be increased up to 1/2 teaspoon per day. Follow the suggested schedule of three weeks on and one week off (during the time of menstruation, if applicable).

Perimenopause

Perimenopausal women often experience the signs and symptoms of estrogen dominance. These include water retention, headaches or migraines, fatigue, breast swelling, fibrocystic breasts, depression or mood swings, loss of sex drive, heavy or irregular menses, uterine fibroids, cravings for sweets, weight gain (particularly around the hips or thighs) and low thyroid symptoms of cold hands and feet.

A perimenopausal woman can follow the generally recommended dosage of natural progesterone. What appears to be the onset of early menopause is often discovered to be estrogen dominance. As progesterone levels increase, the estrogen dominant symptoms will disappear. There is a tendency for doctors to prescribe estrogen if irregular bleeding occurs, however, there is no reason to give estrogen if there is still menstrual bleeding. Menstrual bleeding indicates that there is no estrogen deficiency. Irregular menstrual periods may be the result of low progesterone levels. If you have been put on estrogen for irregular periods, taper down the estrogen and begin using the suggested guidelines for natural progesterone.

It is recommended to use the cream approximately two weeks per month. Between day 12 and day 26 to approximate normal progesterone levels. Some women with longer cycles can take it from day 10 to day 28. If bleeding starts before day 26 (or before it would normally begin), stop using the progesterone. You can then resume using it on day 12. It may take three cycles before normal periods are achieved.

When migraine headaches occur premenstrually, estrogen dominance is often a contributing factor since estrogen dilates the blood vessels. Normal vascular tone is able to restored by using natural progesterone. Natural progesterone can be used ten days before the onset of menstruation. Dr. Lee suggests applying 1/4 to 1/2 teaspoon every three to four hours until the symptoms subside. This usually only necessitates one or two extra applications. He also advises that higher doses of progesterone can be quickly attained with sublingual drops which are more rapidly absorbed than skin cream.

PMS

To use for PMS, follow the above recommendations. However, if you experience cramping or other symptoms during menstruation, you may apply the cream until the symptoms dissipate. The cream can be rubbed on to the lower abdomen during menstrual cramping. If you have migraines during your cycles, the cream can be rubbed on to the back of your neck or on your temples.

As time goes by and the symptoms diminish, try cutting back each month on the amount of natural progesterone you use. If symptoms return, resume the previous dosage. Ultimately, your goal is to be hormonally balanced and symptom free. If you have no symptoms for several months and then symptoms recur, you may want to use the cream as needed. The best way to know if enough is being used is if your symptoms are relieved.

Chapter 16

Natural Estrogens — The Good Guys

Specific plants contain compounds that mimic the actions of estrogen or that favorably affect estrogen metabolism in some way. Although they are considered to be extremely weak compared with human hormones, when used in the diet or in specific natural remedies, they can alleviate menopausal symptoms.

These plant derived estrogens, known as phytoestrogens, are present in a wide variety of foods and herbs. If a woman has an excessive amount of estrogen, these substances help to block the estrogen from entering the estrogen receptor sites. If there is not enough estrogen, they fill the gap. When beneficial phytoestrogens bind to receptor sites, they cannot only supply an alternative form of natural estrogen where needed but by taking up estrogen sites, they may protect the woman from environmental xeno-estrogens which are continually trying to key into those sites.

Phytoestrogens appear to block the effects of excess estrogen stimulation in organs such as the breast and uterus and well may be protective. A particularly rich source of phytoestrogens is found in soy products such as tofu, tempeh, soya milk and miso. One study of Japanese women suggested that a high intake of these products was the reason why they had so few hot flashes or other menopausal symptoms as well as low rates of breast cancer.

An incomplete list of other foods rich in phytoestrogens

includes cashews, peanuts, oats, corn, wheat, apples, almonds, rye, lentils, French beans and pomegranates. Obviously it is essential to eat a diet rich in these foods.

Phytoestrogens have been a part of natural remedies for women's hormonal problems for hundreds of years, if not longer. Herbs used in women's formulas included black cohosh, alfalfa, licorice, red clover and sage. Black cohosh has been known to be a popular herb used by the Native Americans for female complaints.

Estriol — The Underestimated Estrogen

Estriol, along with progesterone, is the estrogen that is made in large quantities during pregnancy. It is made by the placenta. These two main pregnancy sex hormones have potential protective properties against the production of cancerous cells. Estradiol, on the other hand is 1,000 times more potent on breast tissue than estriol. It is well documented that overexposure to estradiol, and to a lesser extent estrone, increases a woman's risk of breast cancer, whereas estriol is protective.[1]

An important 1966 *Journal of American Medical Association* article by H.M. Lemon, M.D., reported a study showing that higher levels of estriol in the body correlate with remission of breast cancer. He showed that women with breast cancer had reduced urinary excretion of estriol. He also observed that women without breast cancer have naturally high levels of estriol and that these women are at much lower risk of breast cancer than other women. Estriol's anti-cancer effect is due to its ability to block the stimulating effects of the other estrogens by blocking the estrogen receptor sites on breast cells.[2]

In fact, A. H. Follingstad, M.D., presented results in *The New England Journal of Medicine* of a study in which small doses of estriol were given to a group of post-menopausal women with spreading breast cancer. An impressive 37 percent of them experienced a remission or arrest of their metastatic lesions. There have been reports that it is better than tamoxifen for women with breast cancer.[3]

Estriol is the estrogen most beneficial to the vagina, cervix and vulva. In cases of postmenopausal vaginal dryness and atrophy which predisposes a woman to vaginitis and cystitis, estriol supplementation would be the most effective and safest estrogen to use. It is also an effective treatment for urinary tract infections.[4]

In addition, estriol, has benefits similar to that of the stronger estrogens but without the risks. It not only reduces menopausal symptoms but increases cardiac function with improved blood flow to the extremities.

Estriol treatment also results in the re-emergence of friendly lactobacilli bacteria and the near elimination of pathologic colon bacteria.

While estriol offers so many benefits to women's health, like natural progesterone, it cannot be patented. It already has established an excellent safety record through its proven track record in Europe as both a prescription drug and an over-the-counter product. Once again, the influence of the pharmaceutical companies and the reluctance of doctors to investigate safe alternatives, restricts a woman's safe and effective options.

While HRT is generally recommended to provide a source of estrogen for women after having a hysterectomy, natural herbal remedies containing phytoestrogens, herbs as well as supplementation with estriol, in addition to natural progesterone, can provide adequate levels of hormones, making HRT unnecessary. If a woman has been eating a healthy diet with abundant amounts of phytoestrogen-rich foods, there is usually adequate estrogen available to her from other estrogen sites in her body such as body fat. After a hysterectomy, it is always advisable to receive advice and guidance from health professionals. Contrary to popular opinion, however, a hysterectomy does not automatically mean a woman must go on HRT for the rest of her life.

Chapter 17

The Relationship Between Hormonal Imbalance and Disease

Exposing the Myths

HRT is now almost universally recommended to menopausal women for a wide variety of reasons. The most significant reasons women are encouraged to embark upon the HRT band wagon are HRT's supposed contribution in preventing or lessening the effects of osteoporosis, cardiovascular disease and more recently, Alzheimer's disease. The tremendous fear of these illnesses that is instilled in patients by well-meaning doctors who, after all, are the targets of effective pharmaceutical advertising and education (usually the only source of information they receive about these products) often over-rides a woman's natural instincts. It's time to unravel the myths that hide the real story.

Osteoporosis

Dr. John Lee, writes the following about the myths of osteoporosis:

Osteoporosis Myth #1
Osteoporosis is a calcium deficiency disease.

Most women with osteoporosis are getting plenty of

calcium in their diet. It is quite easy to get the minimum daily requirement of calcium in even a relatively poor diet. The truth is that osteoporosis is a disease of excessive calcium loss caused by many factors. In osteoporosis, calcium is being lost from the bones faster than it is being added, regardless of how much calcium a woman consumes.

Osteoporosis Myth #2
Osteoporosis is an estrogen deficiency disease.

Not even basic medical texts agree with this—it is a fabrication of the pharmaceutical industry with no scientific evidence to support it. Osteoporosis begins long before estrogen levels fall and accelerates for a few years at menopause. Taking estrogen can slow bone loss for those few years, but its effect wears off within a few years after menopause. Most importantly, estrogen cannot rebuild new bone.

Osteoporosis Myth #3
Osteoporosis is a disease of menopause.

This is at least a decade short of the truth. Osteoporosis begins anywhere from five to 20 years prior to menopause when estrogen levels are still high. Osteoporosis accelerates at menopause or when a woman's ovaries are surgically removed or become non-functional, such as can happen after a hysterectomy. It is staggering to think how many thousands or millions of women have been doomed to a crippled old age and early death because their ovaries and/or uterus were unnecessarily removed before menopause and natural progesterone replacement ignored.

To understand osteoporosis it is important to know a bit about bones. Bone forming cells are of two different kinds. One type are called osteoclasts and their job is to travel through the bone in search of old bone that is in need of renewal. Osteoclasts dissolve bone and leave behind tiny unfilled spaces. Osteoblasts move into these spaces in order to build new bone.

A lack of estrogen as experienced at menopause indirectly stimulates the growth of osteoclasts, increasing the risk for developing osteoporosis. HRT containing estrogen should therefore help prevent osteoporosis. From this point of view, it does.

While osteoclast cells have been shown to have estrogen receptor sites, osteoblast cells, which are responsible for making new bone, have been shown to have, not estrogen, but progesterone receptors. What this means is that it is progesterone (the natural form, not the synthetic progestins) not estrogen which is responsible for building bone tissue.

This view is upheld in *Scientific American's* updated medicine report text, 1991, which states, "Estrogens decrease bone resorption but associated with the decrease in bone resorption is a decrease in bone formation. Therefore, estrogen should not be expected to increase bone mass." The authors also discuss estrogen's side effects, including the risk of endometrial cancer which "is increased six-fold in women who receive estrogen therapy for up to five years; the risk is increased to 15-fold in long term users." So, while estrogen has been shown to slow bone loss in women, it does not arrest it and, in fact, can contribute to other serious health problems.

Slowing down bone loss is in no way the same as building up bone mass. Not only does the use of estrogen for osteoporosis have only a partial effect but what effect it does have is not necessarily permanent. One group of researchers found that within four years of discontinuing estrogen, there was no detectable difference in bone mineral content between women who had never taken the drug and those who began treatment but gave it up. Other studies have shown that six years into menopause estrogen may stop being effective.[1,2]

Dr. Kitty Little from Oxford found masses of tiny clots in the bones of rabbits treated with hormones. She is convinced that HRT, in the form of estrogen and progestins, will increase the risk of osteoporosis. Blood clots originate from sticky clumps of platelet cells in the blood. She believes that blood clots in the bones can cause bone to break down, leading to osteoporosis.[3]

The early studies on which the estrogen-protection assumptions were based had gross scientific defects. Dr. Jerilynn C. Prior, and her colleagues, reporting in the *New England Journal of Medicine*, confirmed that estrogen's role in combating osteoporosis is only a minor one. In their studies of female athletes, they found that osteoporosis occurs to the degree that they become progesterone deficient, even though their estrogen levels seemed to remain normal. [4]

Dr. Prior continued her research with non-athletic women. They showed the same results. While both these groups of women were menstruating, they had anovulatory cycles and were, therefore, progesterone deficient. Dr. Prior then went on to discover that anovulation and a short phase cycle now occurs in up to 50 percent of North American women's menstrual cycles during the final reproductive years. Unfortunately these major findings went relatively unnoticed in the medical community.

As a result of her extensive review of published scientific evidence in this area, Dr. Prior confirmed that it is not estrogen but progesterone which is the bone tropic hormone—that is, the bone builder. They were even able to identify progesterone receptor sites on osteoblast cells (bone tissue building cells). Nobody has ever found osteoblast receptors for estrogen. The bottom line is that it is in women with progesterone deficiency that bone loss occurs. [5]

More and more research findings are emerging that challenge the estrogen deficiency/osteoporosis relationship and reinforce the progesterone deficiency link. The results from a three year study of 63 post-menopausal women with osteoporosis verify this. Women using transdermal progesterone cream experienced an average 7-8 percent bone mass density increase in the first year, 4-5 percent the second year and 3-4 percent the third year. Untreated women in this age category typically lose 1.5 percent bone mass density per year! These results have not been found with any other form of hormone replacement therapy or dietary supplementation. [6]

Dr. Margaret Smith, a specialist in medical gynecology and medical founder of the first menopause clinic in Western

Australia, believes that, "In the next five years we are going to find that natural progesterone is going to replace or displace all the progestins because it will be shown to be that much more effective in actually restoring bone loss, not just preventing bone loss, as well as making women feel well."

Despite this clear evidence of the importance of progesterone to bone formation, very little attention has been given to it by the medical establishment. Dr. William Regelson, a leading researcher in hormones and the author of *The Super-Hormone Promise*, flatly states, "Given the fact that 25 percent of all women are at risk of developing osteoporosis, I think it is unconscionable that progesterone's role in this disease has been neglected."[7]

Another intriguing fact sheds serious doubt on estrogen's key role in bone health. Studies using tamoxifen which is an anti-estrogen drug given to breast cancer prone women to block the uptake of estrogen hormones have shown no bone loss in women. If lack of estrogen is the cause of osteoporosis, tamoxifen would have caused significant bone density loss.[8]

Bone loss is the result of many other factors besides progesterone deficiency. Excess protein in the form of meat and dairy products (contrary to the dairy industry's advertising) contribute to bone loss. An acidic condition is created in the blood which then causes the body to extract calcium from the bones to neutralize it. Another major factor is lack of exercise. Bone growth is dependent on weight bearing exercise. In addition, sugar, diuretics, antibiotics, inadequate levels of hydrochloric acid in the stomach, caffeine, fluoride, cigarettes, alcohol abuse and cortisone all are deleterious to bones.

There is a huge amount of confusion about the place of calcium supplements as a safeguard against osteoporosis. It seems, in fact, that calcium supplements are raising some concern. *Lunar News* (December 1994) reported, "it is unclear why the risk of hip fracture is doubled by high calcium." Another study showed that calcium supplementation in adults, normal elderly subjects or the osteoporotic, had little effect (less than

4 percent increase) on bones, but it did increase constipation and flatulence (more than 10 percent).[9]

The best source of calcium is from calcium-rich foods which include sardines, canned salmon, dark green leafy vegetables, Brazil nuts, tofu and all soy products, sunflower seeds and hulled sesame seeds.

In summary, post menopausal osteoporosis is a disease of excess bone loss caused primarily by a progesterone deficiency and secondarily by poor diet, nutritional deficiencies and lack of adequate weight bearing exercise. While progesterone assists in the restoration of bone mass and is an essential factor in the prevention and proper treatment of osteoporosis at any age, it should be considered as one of several key ingredients in bone health.[10] Bone building is a chain of linked factors each of which must be strong for the chain to be strong.

Cardiovascular Disease

Estrogen is being touted by mainstream medicine as a great preventive of cardiovascular disease in women and therefore a major reason to have women on HRT. To understand the issues at hand, it is first important to understand just what is cardiovascular disease. Cardiovascular disease incudes both heart disease and stroke. Stroke, like heart disease, is a vascular disease: a disease of blood vessels. In both cases the blood vessels become narrow either through spasm or through atherosclerosis, the narrowing of the arteries that feed the heart. Therefore not enough blood gets to a critical place. In the case of heart disease it is the heart and with strokes it is to the brain. Cardiovascular disease also encompasses high blood pressure and coronary artery disease.

Dr. Susan Love says, "Heart disease is not a symptom of menopause. Heart disease is heart disease. It's more common in postmenopausal women that in pre-menopausal women but that's because postmenopausal women are older than pre-menopausal women. It's like gray hair; you're more likely to have gray hair after menopause than before it but menopause doesn't cause gray hair—rather, they both tend to happen in later life.

"The standard line has always been that women are protected from heart disease as long as their bodies make estrogen, and then after menopause they lose that protection and the rates of heart disease for men and women become equal. But in fact, the rates never become equal. In this country, women in their sixties and seventies have 45 percent less heart disease than men in the same age bracket. Women develop heart disease much later than men— seven or eight years later. Women's risk rises continuously as they get older but there's no sudden increase with menopause. We never catch up."[11]

It is interesting to note that the *Physicians' Desk Reference* warns that women should not take estrogen or progestins if they have current or past clotting disorders, thrombosis, a stroke history, cerebrovascular or cardiovascular disorders, high lipoproteins (a specific type of blood fats), severe uncontrolled hypertension or lipid metabolism disorders. In addition, cigarette smoking increases the risk of serious cardiovascular effects from the use of estrogens.

It is also an undisputed fact that estrogen and progestins, the two key ingredients of oral contraceptives, have been responsible for strokes, blood clots and heart attacks in women taking The Pill.

Estrogen does appear to lower total cholesterol and raise HDL cholesterol (the good one) modestly. However, it is no where conclusive that this reduces the risk of heart mortality per se. Significant new findings also show that natural progesterone has the same effect.

In light of these known risks, it is certainly curious that estrogen and the use of HRT is so rigorously pursued by the pharmaceutical companies and the medical profession as a treatment for the prevention of cardiovascular disease.

According to Dr. Lee, the one notable study which formed the entire basis of the positive estrogen-cardiovascular link, the 1991 *New England Journal of Medicine* report known as the *Boston Nurses' Questionnaire Study* (conducted using a large sampling

of nurses), was radically flawed and the statistics manipulated.[12] Although there is ample evidence from numerous other
studies showing that, indeed, the opposite is true—estrogen
is a significant factor in creating heart disease—these findings
have been virtually ignored in the frenzy for profits. Dr. Lee
goes on to say that pharmaceutical advertisements neglected
to mention the fact that stroke death incidence from that study
was 50 percent higher among the estrogen users.

In 1985, another notable study, the Framingham Heart
Study, the only ongoing, long-term epidemiological study in
the United States conducted on 240,000 women reported that
their postmenopausal estrogen users had no increased incidence of heart disease but a 50 percent increase in strokes as
non-estrogen users. Estrogen users had a higher risk of vascular
disease which was independent of other main known risks
such as early menopause.[13] Their conclusion was that there is
no coronary benefit from estrogen use. In fact, other studies
have found increased cardiovascular disease risk from estrogen use. In her *New England Journal of Medicine* letter to editor,
following the publication of the *Boston Nurses Questionnaire
Study*, Dr. Jerilynn C. Prior listed 16 references disputing the
claim that estrogen provided cardiovascular benefit.

Alarming evidence has recently surfaced from animal studies which demonstrates that synthetic progestins (Provera)
co-administered with estrogen counteracts any beneficial
effects estrogen may have in preventing heart disease and
stroke. It actually was found to increase the risk of coronary
vasospasms, narrowing of arteries to the heart that can lead
to a heart attack.[14]

While researching the estrogen-cardiovascular link Nancy
Beckham found the following:[15]

❖ High doses of estrogens are likely to be thrombo-
   genic (blood clotting) during use and it is possible
   that even moderate doses may increase the risk
   of clotting among women who smoke or who
   already have clogged arteries. Reports are now

starting to come in indicating that high-dose estrogens, particularly as experienced with estradiol implants, cause hyper-coagulability, which means that the blood has a tendency to clot, thereby increasing the risk of heart attacks and stroke.

❖ A British medical report also states that the cardiovascular effects of synthetic progestins used with estrogen in the much larger number of women who have not undergone hysterectomy are unknown.

❖ Some researchers do not consider that heart disease is linked to the cessation of the body's estrogen production. (Actually it is inaccurate to use the word 'cessation' since estrogen production is only reduced in menopause.)

Natural progesterone seems to play a significant role in protecting women from cardiovascular disease. We know now that anovulatory cycles and lowered progesterone levels occur prior to menopause; and progesterone levels after menopause are close to zero. Estrogen, on the other hand, falls only 40-60 percent with menopause. A woman's passage through menopause results in a greater loss of progesterone than of estrogen. Perhaps the increased risk of heart disease after menopause is due more to progesterone deficiency than to estrogen deficiency. Dr. Lee has noted in his clinical experience that lipid profiles improve when progesterone is supplemented.[16]

In an interview published by the American Medical Association on the Internet, Dr. Elizabeth Barrett-Connor remarked, "If I were treating a woman primarily because she had dyslipidemia (abnormal blood fats) and low HDL cholesterol, I would probably see if she wanted to take micronized progesterone. I was quite impressed with the better effect." What is known about progesterone is that it increases the burning of fats for energy and has an anti-inflammatory effect. Both of these actions could be protective against coronary heart disease. Progesterone protects the integrity and function of cell membranes, whereas estrogen allows the influx of sodium and water while allowing the loss of potassium and magnesium. Progesterone, a natural diuretic, promotes better sleep patterns and helps lessen stress. When one reviews the known actions of progesterone, it is clear that many of its actions are also beneficial to the heart.

When it comes to increased risks of coronary disease, dietary factors are extremely important. Heart disease risk is increased by the following: general overeating, transfatty acids, animal fats, sugars and refined carbohydrates, over-processed foods, excess salt or sodium, lack of fiber, magnesium and/or potassium deficiency and lack of anti-oxidant rich food or supplements such as vitamins C, E, A, beta-carotene, folate and selenium. Stress is also a major risk factor for heart disease.

Cardiovascular disease would be much more effectively treated if more attention was placed on its many contributing factors. According to Dr. Graham Colditz, Harvard professor and project director of the *Boston Nurses Questionnaire Study* the known breast cancer risk for women from estrogen is of such concern that other more effective treatment and life style approaches should be the first line of defense. They include: stop smoking, exercise, Vitamin E and folate, weight reduction and dietary changes.

The observations of Dr. Elizabeth Barret-Connor were written in a paper in 1993. She stated, "No other prescription drug has been given on such a large scale to prevent disease in healthy women without proof of efficacy by a randomized clinical trial. It is also important to remember that estrogen replacement is drug treatment, not really replacement therapy; the dose and route are unphysiologic and the level of circulating estrone is higher than sustained by pre-menopausal women."[17]

Hormones and Cancer

The evidence connecting female cancers of the breast, uterus and ovaries with high estrogen levels is growing. Estrogen's job in the uterus is to cause proliferation of the cells. Under the influence of estrogen, uterine cells multiply faster, then progesterone normally should be released at ovulation and stop the cells from multiplying. Progesterone causes the cells to mature and enter the secretory phase that causes the maturing of the uterine lining, which is now ready to receive a possible fertilized egg. Estrogen is the hormone that stimulates cell proliferation and progesterone is the hormone that stops growth and stimulates ripening.

Breast Cancer

Estrogen dominance also stimulates breast tissue: premenstrual women who suffer from estrogen dominance often suffer from breast swelling and tenderness. Progesterone, as a hormone of maturation, brings the cells back into balance and thus can eliminate breast tenderness.

There is certainly an alarmingly high incidence of breast and uterine cancer amongst western women. There is evidence that breast cancer occurs most often at the stage of life when estrogen is dominant for the full month and progesterone is not coming in ovulation—the halfway point. Dr. Graham Colditz, maintains that the use of unopposed estrogen for 10 years or more is responsible for 30-40 percent of breast cancers. However, women who took estrogen plus progesterone increased their risk by up to 100 percent[18]

Johns Hopkins Private Obstetrics and Gynecology Clinic accumulated 40 years of research which was published in the *American Journal of Epidemiology* in 1981.[19] What they discovered was that when the low progesterone group was compared to the normal progesterone group, it was found that the occurrence of breast cancer was 5.4 times greater in the women in the low progesterone group. That is, the incidence of breast cancer in the low progesterone group was over 80 percent greater than in the normal progesterone group.

When the study looked at the low progesterone group for all types of cancer, they found that women in the low progesterone group experienced a tenfold increase from all malignant cancers, compared to the normal progesterone group. This would suggest that having a normal level of progesterone protected women from nine-tenths of all cancers that might otherwise have occurred. It is interesting to note that the study disappeared into oblivion when there was no money available to pursue the obvious implications of a progesterone deficiency role in cancer.

In a 1995 study published in the *Journal of Fertility and Sterility*, researchers did a double-blind randomized study examining the use of topical progesterone cream and/or topical estrogen in regard to breast cell growth. The result showed that women using progesterone had dramatically reduced cell multiplication rates compared to the women using either the placebo or estrogen. The women using only estrogen had significantly higher cell multiplication rates than any of the other groups, The women using a combination of progesterone and estrogen were closer to the placebo group.[20]

This exciting study provides some of the first direct evidence that estradiol significantly increases breast cell growth and that progesterone impressively decreases cell proliferation rates, even when estrogen is also supplemented.

It has also been shown that among premenopausal women, breast cancer recurrence or late metastases after mastectomy, was more common when surgery had been performed during the first half of the menstrual cycle, when estrogen is the dominant hormone, than when surgery had been performed during the progesterone dominant latter half of the menstrual cycle.

Recently there have been disturbing studies about still another possible effect of hormone therapy on the risk of breast cancer. This has to do with the effects of HRT on breast tissue. HRT can stimulate breast tissue causing it to become more dense. Cancer and breast tissue are the same density, so a mammogram can give false readings. Researchers at the University of Washington looked at the records of 8,779 postmenopausal women who had mammograms for breast cancer. Women on estrogen had 33 percent more false positives (showing an abnormality but none could be found) and 423 percent more false negatives (an abnormality was missed that showed up later) than women not using estrogen.[21]

Tamoxifen — Beware

At this point, it is important to explore the implications of the experimental drug tamoxifen, a synthetic hormone similar in structure to DES which has been prescribed to more than three million women with breast cancer since 1970. Since it is purported to have anti-estrogenic effects it is used as a breast cancer treatment, blocking the uptake of estradiol and estrone (the cell proliferating estrogens) and thereby protecting the breast tissue from the cancer-promoting estrogens present in the body. Among the choices of orthodox medicine, it certainly is the kinder treatment compared with chemotherapy, radiotherapy or surgery.

However, tamoxifen is not without its dangers. It is a known carcinogen. One study showed that 27 percent of women taking tamoxifen showed hyperplastic (unfavorable new growth) changes in their wombs within fifteen months.[22] Taking 20mg of tamoxifen per day can increase the risk of developing uterine cancer by up to five times.

In addition, eye damage, retinopathy, has been reported in seven percent of women in one study, while menopausal symptoms such as hot flashes, vaginal discharge or dryness, irregular menses, nausea and depression are the most common side-effects. Thrombombolic disease (a clotting disorder) is seven times more frequent. According to Dr. Susan Love, when it's taken for a year, tamoxifen increases bone loss in premenopausal women though it does prevent further bone loss in postmenopausal women.

Dr. Susan Love also reports that, "there is reason to believe that even tamoxifen's supposed role in preventing breast cancer should be questioned. Earlier studies had shown that when women who had cancer in one breast took tamoxifen, it reduced the risk of cancer in the other breast by 30-50 percent. A more recent randomized controlled study, however, showed that it had its maximum effect with women who took it for five years. Taking it for five more years didn't offer any more protection and may actually have caused more cancers, In other words, after a while the breast cells become resistant to tamoxifen and actually start to be fed by it."[23]

One study showed just a meagre 0.7 percent benefit for women taking Tamoxifen preventively to reduce the risk of developing further tumors in the breast.[24] To make matters worse, Dr. Ellen Grant, author of *Sexual Chemistry*, has reported that in tamoxifen treated subjects, new tumors that do appear tend to be highly malignant with an increased mortality.

While a known carcinogen, the *Science News* (March 2, 1996) reported rather shocking information about tamoxifen. The World Health Organization (WHO) has formally designated tamoxifen as a human carcinogen, grouping it with roughly 70 other chemicals, about one-quarter of them pharmaceuticals that have received this dubious distinction.[25]

However, there are safer alternatives to tamoxifen. One of the estrogens produced by the ovaries is called estriol (weaker than the other two, estradiol and estrone). Estriol is considered a safe estrogen in that it has been shown to inhibit breast cancer. Dr. Henry Lemon and his colleagues conducted a study in women who already had breast cancer that had spread to other areas of the body. One group was given estriol and another not. At the end of the study, 37 percent of those women who received estriol had either a remission or an arrest of their cancer.[26] Might not estriol, a natural, safe hormone with almost no side effects, be able to accomplish what tamoxifen does but without the toxic side-effects?

A growing number of doctors also insist that the same results can be achieved by giving natural progesterone.

It is also interesting to note that menstruating women who have breast surgery carried out during the second half of their menstrual cycle—the luteal phase when progesterone is high to balance estrogens—survive far longer than do women whose surgery is done early in their cycle, during the estrogen-dominant follicular phase.[27]

Endometrial Cancer

The only known cause of endometrial cancer is unopposed estrogen. Here again the culprits are estradiol and estrone. Estrogen supplements given to postmenopausal women for five years increase the risk of endometrial cancer sixfold and longer-term use increases it 15-fold. In perimenopausal women, endometrial cancer is extremely rare except during the five to ten years before menopause when estrogen dominance is common.[28]

Cervical Cancer

Synthetic hormones are also linked to cervical cancer. The cells of the cervix are extremely hormone-sensitive. Levels of synthetic progestins, low enough not to alter the cells of the lining of the womb, have been shown to change the cells that line the cervix. Progestins dry up cervical secretions and this may be part of the reason why cancer of the cervix develops quickly in the presence of cervical infections.[29]

Ovarian Cancer

On May 1, 1995, the American Cancer Society announced further alarming statistics from a study of ERT and ovarian cancer. It showed that among the 240,000 postmenopausal women who had no prior history of cancer, hysterectomy or ovarian surgery. Participating in this 13 year prospective mortality study, the risk of fatal ovarian cancer was 40 percent higher for women who used estrogen for at least 6 years and 70 percent higher at 11 years of use. The obvious conclusion from the study was that long-term use of estrogen replacement therapy may increase the risk of fatal ovarian cancer.[30]

Melanomas

It was predicted in the 1960's that the Pill would increase the chances of a woman developing a melanoma, the most lethal of all skin cancers. Hormones control the pigmentation of our skin and melanoma cancer cells have estrogen receptors which can make the growth of cancer more likely. Women taking the Pill and HRT are at greater risk in developing melanomas than the average woman.

In animal tests, estrogen stimulates the formation of the black pigment melanin but the effect is greatly augmented by the addition of a progestin—as in the Pill. Because hormones control pigmentation, the early researchers thought that oral contraceptives would predispose to the development of malignant melanomas.[31] The tumors, like breast cancer cells have estrogen receptors and women on HRT are also more likely to develop melanomas.

The Walnut Creek study found Pill and HRT users were more likely to develop melanomas. All the women who developed melanomas under age forty had taken the Pill. By 1981, the overall increased risk for ever-users was statistically significant at three times.[32]

An Australian case-control study described how more than five years of pill use significantly increased the melanoma risk if the pill had been started ten years before the cancer was diagnosed. The increase remained significant even after adjustment for many factors. The study found increases among women who had been given hormones to regulate their periods, as HRT or to suppress lactation.[33]

Alzheimer's Disease

Just the mention of Alzheimer's strikes fear in the heart of people. Nothing seems to be as devastating as the loss of mental faculties. While the medical profession has given Alzheimer's disease a rather high profile these days, it actually isn't all that common. It is also more likely to affect the very old. It's 14 times more common in people over the age of 85 than in those between 60 and 65 years of age. It seems that women have 1.5 to 3 times more risk of getting Alzheimer's than men which may, in part, simply be because women live longer.[34]

A theory has been suggested that estrogen may protect against Alzheimer's disease. As is so often the case with synthetic hormones, an hypothesis has been quickly transformed into unsubstantiated fact.

The study that gave credence to this theory was published in the *American Journal of Epidemiology* in 1994. The study was based upon a group of 127 postmenopausal residents in a retirement community in California called Leisure World. Investigators compared the women whose death certificates mentioned Alzheimer's or dementia with the matched record of decedents who hadn't died of either cause. They found that estrogen users were 30 percent less likely than non-users to have died of either condition. The researchers also found that Alzheimer's patients on estrogen performed better on a standard mental exam than patients who weren't.[35] The researchers of the study believe that it hints at a possible connection but research is far from conclusive.

It is important to remember that in the world of medical research and clinical trials there are usually conflicting data and results. So, it comes as no surprise that in a quite similar study involving residents of Rancho Bernardo, California, women decedents who had taken estrogen were found to be almost twice as likely to have died of Alzheimer's disease as women who had never taken it. Further, when the researchers compared the test scores for memory and mental acuity of the users and never-users, no significant differences were found.[36]

While inconclusive as well as conflicting results about the estrogen-Alzheimer link compete for medical and public attention, the pharmaceutical companies along with medical establishment are jumping the gun on estrogen's benefits on the brain. Dr. Love reported that one of Wyeth-Ayerst's representatives (the manufacture of Premarin) announced at a conference on hormones that "cognition can provide the gut-level response to breast cancer." The implication was that if the makers of Premarin could show that estrogen prevents Alzheimer's disease, it would be enough of a benefit to counteract women's fear of getting breast cancer from taking estrogen: fear of Alzheimer's trumps fear of breast cancer.[37]

Once again, sensational advertising campaigns can successfully masquerade as factual medical science.

Chapter 18

Men and Natural Progesterone

Present research confirms that men can also benefit from natural progesterone. In men, progesterone is synthesized by their testes to produce testosterone and in their adrenals to produce corticosteroids. In fact, the prostate gland has specific progesterone receptor sites. Healthy men continue to produce normal testosterone and corticosteroid levels into their seventies and eighties.

Men also make the estrogen, estradiol, but in much lower amounts than women. Testosterone, like progesterone, is an antagonist to estradiol. Testosterone prevents estradiol from causing prostate cancer by destroying the prostate cancer cells which estrogen stimulates.

The prostate is the male equivalent of the uterus since they both develop from the same embryonic cells, thus also being affected by exposure to excess estrogens, endogenously or exogenously.

As men age, progesterone levels decrease just as they do in women. For most women, this decrease occurs around the age of 35. In men it occur 10 years later. When progesterone levels decrease, an enzyme called 5 alpha reductase is then able to convert testosterone to another type of testosterone known as dihydrotestosterone (DHT). Research is discovering that it is the DHT content in the prostate which is the single most causative factor in prostate disease, not testosterone, itself.

Studies have shown that progesterone inhibited estrogen from binding to the prostate, inhibited the formation and binding of DHT and reduced 5-alpha reductase activity, In test animals, progesterone reduced the prostate of test animals.

Estradiol also stimulates the enlargement of the prostate. When the prostate gland swells and enlarges, it is called benign prostatic hyperplasia (BHP). This condition causes the need to urinate more frequently and urinary incontinence. Progesterone has shown to be even more effective in inhibiting 5 alpha reductase than either Proscar or Saw Palmetto.

Estrogen levels increase in again men who are overweight because fat cells convert the male hormone androstenedione into estrogens which stimulates prostate growth. Thus, an overweight man will have higher estradiol levels. Estrogen dominant symptoms such as weight gain, enlarged breasts, gall bladder problems, anxiety and insomnia also occur in men.

The amount of progesterone made by men is 4-6 mg. per day. Men can take progesterone daily without taking any time off. It is suggested that men take 5 mg (1/16 tsp) twice daily, applying it to the scrotum. It has also been recommended to use a low dose (4-6 mg.) of natural testosterone from a cream or patch. Maintaining a healthy prostate also involves other factors such as diet, specific nutrients, herbs, essential fatty acids, antioxidants and stress management. As with all symptoms of hormonal imbalance and dysfunction, it is crucial to consult with a qualified holistic practitioner.

Hormonal balance is the key to male hormonal health. Balance is more about maintaining the proper ratio of hormones rather than absolute concentration levels of any one hormone. It is the ratio of salivary concentrations of testosterone to estradiol that best reflects the hormone-related risk of prostate cancer. Thus, saliva testing is also an important diagnostic and predictive tool for assessing men's hormone levels. Using a combination of natural hormone approaches along with dietary and lifestyle changes would seem a much more sensible approach to prostate health and prostate cancer treatment than castration, radiation or prostatectomy. These conventional approaches can cause impotence, incontinence, and bowel, stomach and rectal problems.

For those men who have already been chemically or surgically castrated from their prostate treatment and are at high risk of osteoporosis, Dr. Lee has found that, "If one wishes to prevent or treat the castration-induced osteoporosis, it is possible to safely supplement progesterone to replace testosterone in these men."[1]

A personal account from a contributing doctor to the guidebook, *Alternative Medicine: The Definitive Guide* confirms a similar experience. "Topical application of natural progesterone may prove beneficial in the treatment of prostate conditions. The doctor reports working with twelve men, all in their late seventies, who were suffering from osteoporosis. As it has been well established that natural progesterone applied topically can relieve osteoporosis, the physician suggested that the men systematically massage it into their skin on a daily basis. All of them began to experience relief from their condition and later called to tell (the doctor) that, after three months, they were also experiencing an improved urine flow, with less pressure on their prostate glands and noticeable decrease in nightly urination."[2]

Dr. Norman Shealey, medical practitioner and author, also believed that natural progesterone benefits men. He began to use natural progesterone on his older male patients. The progesterone apparently caused one patient's DHEA hormone level to double. His libido soared and he felt better than he had in years. In fact. Dr. Shealey discovered that the majority of men who used the natural progesterone cream showed a marked increase (60 to 100 percent) in their DHEA. This is important news, since DHEA seems to spark the metabolism of both men and women and helps balance the entire glandular system. More research on the connection between these two hormones is definitely in order.[3]

It is now being realized that the conventional testosterone hypothesis is a 60-year old mistake. The choices of treatment on offer from traditional medical doctors are debilitating, dangerous and have limited effectiveness. It is obvious that male health problems are not immune to the ignorance that pervades modern medicine.

Chapter 19

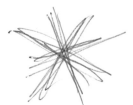

An Integrative Approach

There are a number of ways in which women can attend to the various symptoms and illnesses that hormonal imbalance may be causing. Dietary changes, exercise, naturopathy, chiropractic care, classical osteopathy, acupuncture, homeopathy, Western and Eastern herbal medicine, aromatherapy and stress management techniques are some of the safe and effective options presently available. There isn't necessarily just one way. Having the options to integrate more than one therapy into a woman's preferred choice of treatment provides her with the best of each modality. Doctors and complementary health practitioners can both have their place in a woman's healthcare program. Why not take the best from all possible worlds?

Aside from finding a qualified health practitioner, it is also important to choose someone with whom there is a comfortable rapport. A relationship based upon mutual respect, courtesy and compassion is a truly healing relationship.

Chapter 20

The Challenge Before Us

The hormone story is certainly a very complicated one. Up until now only one version of the story has been available to the majority of Western women. Serious doubt has been cast on the efficacy and appropriateness of estrogen and progestins as the first choice in treatment. Women are certainly suffering more than ever before from a wide variety of female complaints. What complicates the hormone story is that the seeming cures for these complaints may actually make them worse. Without understanding the far-reaching side-effects of estrogen dominance and progestins, doctors are often misdiagnosing the cause of these aggravated conditions. Other drugs may then be prescribed, with disastrous effects, as the spiral of unnecessary medication increases. What is the toll being taken not only to a woman's deteriorating health and emotional well-being but also to her financial situation, her relationships and her career?

Without adequate knowledge, education and access to natural products, women have been easy prey to the powerful campaigns of the multinational drug companies that have convinced doctors and governments of their claims. It is becoming more evident that women's interests are not always best met through such a biased approach. It is not unusual for profits to take precedence over health and well-being. The last thing a woman needs is to have her natural bodily functions denigrated to deficiency diseases which then necessitate ongoing medical attention.

The long road we have been travelling for almost 40 years has encouraged and promoted the wide range of synthetic hormone products and it is taking us to a tragic dead-end. The scare tactic techniques and intimidation employed by doctors and pharmaceutical companies alike to use such products, often over riding a women's better judgment, have pushed millions of women into using drugs that are unproven and unsafe. It is no surprise, therefore, that Dr. Lee has issued an ominous warning when he says, "we will soon regard making estrogen the key ingredient in Hormone Replacement Therapy as a major medical mistake."[1]   Unfortunately, the same can now be said about progestins.

The same message is reiterated by Leslie Kenton in her book *Passage to Power* when she says that "one of the greatest ironies at the turn of the millennium is that for almost half a century women have been encouraged to use estrogens. They have been sold as a means of birth control and for counteracting negative symptoms experienced at menopause. Yet it turns out that excessive estrogen may well be the greatest enemy any woman in the industrialized world ever faces."

Women must be able to make educated, informed choices about their bodies and their health treatment preferences. It's impossible to make important health decisions if fundamental facts are missing or misconstrued. It is also evident that the health care providers we have come to rely upon either have not received adequate, unbiased education themselves or have become imprisoned by their own arrogant and narrow-minded points of view.

According to Dr. Lee, "There is revolution underfoot. The revolution is not driven by doctors. The revolution is being driven by the women. There is probably no better teacher for doctors than a resourceful, assertive, intelligent woman who knows what she is talking about. When she goes to her doctor and says, 'I have tried estrogen, it made me bloat, it made my breasts swell, it made me feel terrible and I couldn't concentrate (and a whole long list of other side-effects) so I decided to go on the progesterone cream and reduce my estrogen and now I am so much better. I want you to follow me in this', remembering that this is the way to carry on the revolution."

It is indeed time for women to take even greater responsibility for their health, their choices and their life-style. The greatest weapon against compliance and ignorance is knowledge. It's time to ask poignant questions of your health provider, to demand answers and to be willing to investigate safe, alternative approaches. It is apparent that women will need to participate in educating their doctors of the other choices that exist as well as the ones that they prefer. It is a woman's right to choose with dignity the best approach to her own health care.

It is up to every woman to read, question, trust her natural instincts and learn about her own body. It is also essential that women honor their own cyclic nature and intuitive wisdom. A woman's body is her ally in her search for health and healing. Listening to the wisdom of her body is the path to self-discovery, joy and well-being.

PART TWO

The Journey to Hell and Back

Women's Personal Stories

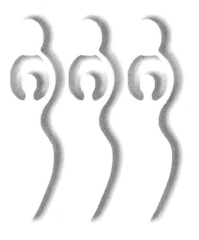

A Personal Perspective

In writing this book, it was first a journey of researching the facts. I sifted through piles of articles, journals, studies and books. As part of this academic exercise, I personally tracked down and interviewed the experts for their opinions on the subject. It was a massive learning experience. I uncovered startling research that seriously challenged the zealous promotion of synthetic hormones' supposed wonders. (Studies that somehow disappeared into oblivion.) I also learned how statistics have been tinkered with and manipulated to give credence to any theory or point of view. Medicine has always been, after all, a battle field for competing hypotheses that rise and fall out of favor on a regular basis. However, facts and stats, as enlightening as they may be, are still intellectual abstractions devoid of the flesh and blood of the human emotional experience.

This book would have been a glorious intellectual exercise if it wasn't for the intimate experiences I had while talking with hundreds and hundreds of women. They spoke of their confusion, physical and emotional pain, despair and anger. It was as though they had become lost in an endless maze of doctors' visits, tests and medications. A maze that always led to another dead end. They also spoke of how their 'Pill' and HRT experience shattered self-esteem, relationships and careers. And that horrible helplessness feeling that comes when you know your health is mysteriously draining away accompanied by the terror when your bodily functions seem to be careening completely out of control.

The following personal journeys are authentic stories from women who unknowingly found their lives to be casualties of synthetic hormones found either in oral contraceptives or HRT. They bravely consented to share their personal experiences as testimonies to the courage, inner wisdom and perseverance that eventually brought them back to health. Their stories are truly inspirational. While they may seem extreme, in fact, women all over the world have been recounting similar experiences. I have heard thousands of variations of the same theme. These are women who were fortunate to find their way out of the synthetic hormone induced darkness. Their collective wish is that their experiences may serve as beacons of light guiding other women safely on their way to greater hormonal health.

Kate's Story

As a 38 year old mother of three, I began to experience hot flushes and cessation of my period two years ago. All the signs indicated early menopause so I promptly consulted a specialist physician who heads a local menopause clinic for women. She prescribed oral estrogen (Premarin) and when this failed to raise my serum levels, she suggested Estraderm patches then finally an estrogen and testosterone implant. Synthetic progestin (Provera) was taken orally from day 14 to 26.

It struck me, while bracing myself against the pain as my GP cut a small incision in my backside, that I'd have to subject myself to this implant procedure every six months for the rest of my life in fear of heart disease or osteoporosis. Without question, pharmaceutical-driven propaganda had successfully convinced me that menopause was indeed a disease and that I could not survive my life cycles without medical intervention.

Ill health had plagued me since the birth of my third child and a tubal ligation in March, 1989. Diffused muscle soreness and stiffness was diagnosed as fibromyalgia that had become so chronic I lived on 2-3 Mercyndol a day. Excessive weight gain (40 lbs.) and loss of energy did little for my libido. Bloating, sleep disturbance, chronic fatigue, incontinence, tender and somewhat lob-sided breasts and migraines all intensified over time. My face became dry and pimply with the added bonus of excessive facial hair.

HRT was introduced to alleviate symptoms, protect against early aging and restore my health.

At no time did I understand exactly (1) why I was on HRT other than it was recommended in the treatment of menopause, (2) what quantifiable gains I could expect or (3) the risks involved.

My inner disquiet spilled over into my relationship with family and friends. I made other people miserable because that's how I felt within myself. I'd become downright aggressive, exhibiting dramatic mood swings that usually ended in a teary apology. Some days the anxiety attacks were so severe I'd climb into bed, pull the covers over my head and wouldn't come up for air all day. Getting through the day was a major feat. I was spiralling down a black hole that swallowed me by degrees every day. And what I feared most was the loss of my loved ones as my growing madness was mirrored in their eyes.

Of course, I tried pouring my heart out to a psychologist but quickly realized he did little more than pull on an already depleted bank account. Certainly, I knew I wasn't insane. It just felt that way most of the time.

May 1996, in preparation for an implant, I was injected with a high dose of estrogen. Even before my physician had removed the syringe, my breasts were stinging. The sensation was not unlike that of a mother's breast filling or 'letting down' with milk during breast-feeding. My GP reassured me it wasn't anything to be concerned about. I figured if she wasn't concerned then everything must be ok! We were both wrong. Four months later a second opinion confirmed a lump in my right breast.

Since offering my body up to HRT over an eighteen month period, I was hospitalized for tests to investigate vaginal bleeding that included a D&C, repair of cervical erosion and cancer screening of the cervix, uterus and breast. Why was my physician so vigilant for cancer? Did HRT involve risks I'd not heard about?

One day, I some how got my tablets mixed up. I mistook a few Premarin tablets for Provera and overdosed on estrogen. My body, already weakened in its struggle with the estrogen implant, could not handle the introduction of this extra estrogen. And what followed made a miscarriage look rather tame. Fifteen days later and still clotting, my doctor prescribed synthetic progestin every two hours until the bleeding came back under control. After this episode of heavy bleeding, I began to seriously contemplate a hysterectomy.

On the assumption my symptoms were directly the result of too much estrogen in my body, I decided to try a natural progesterone cream. I began massaging the cream onto my face, arms, tummy but concentrating on my breasts. Some weeks later, after cancelling my mammogram appointment three times, I finally found the courage to front up for tests. To my utter relief, the results came back all clear. Remarkably, there was no lump to investigate. And if that wasn't irrefutable evidence of the positive effects from natural progesterone, I also began menstruating again naturally.

Initially my menstrual flow was heavy with excessive clotting. Nonetheless, over a matter of months my period took on a regular, more natural cycle. Natural progesterone appeared to have a positive impact on estrogen's known side effect—thickening of the endometrium.

These days I'm up out of bed around 5:00 am most mornings and rarely do I reach for a Panadol. I no longer suffer from fibromyalgia, incontinence or fibrocystic breasts. My energy levels and libido have returned and my weight has stabilized. For the first time in my reproductive life I can chart my menstrual cycle on a calendar!

Whatever my condition one thing is for certain, natural progesterone restored my health where prescription drugs could not. I concluded that the much publicized HRT debate is not about what the doctors or pharmaceutical companies claim will or should work in my body. It's about making an informed choice and having access to ALL the facts and remedies, both orthodox and complementary. After all, I am the walking, talking laboratory animal on whom these drugs are tested.

Franka's Story

As I look back at the last twelve years of my life, I can only but give thanks that I am still alive today. At 51 years of age and a psychologist with a successful practice, I am only now beginning to recover my physical and psychological health from my descent into the hell that HRT caused me. Of course, for all that time I had no idea that the very hormone drugs I was being prescribed were actually responsible for my deteriorating condition.

It all began at the age of 38 when I became aware of increasing hot flashes, leg cramps, dizziness and extreme mood swings. My GP diagnosed me as having an early menopause and prescribed Premarin. I stayed on that medication for the next six years.

However, over that time my symptoms continued to worsen. My gynecologist at that time decided to change my medication to 1.25 mg. of Ogen with Provera for tens days of the month. I was told to take three tablets of Ogen daily. For a brief time I thought the HRT was working as my hot flashes, leg cramps and mood swings seemed to stabilize. But it was only temporary and before very long my symptoms and a whole host of others returned with a vengeance.

My emotions would seesaw from violent outbursts of anger and rage to uncontrollable weeping. I became increasingly more depressed and anxious, finding myself obsessing with worry over the smallest things. I had found myself transformed from a very positive and optimistic person to one who had to struggle to find anything good in a situation. I was getting more and more critical, especially with my family members. I fought with my daughter, actually coming to blows with her once—something that I had never done my whole life. My life really descended to the depths when I decided to separate from my husband of over twenty years. I was constantly critical and angry with him. He could do nothing right in my eyes. Through all this, my self-esteem was eroding away.

Riding this extreme roller coaster of emotions made me feel as though I was possessed. At the time, I didn't put any of these symptoms down to the HRT, I just thought that I was going crazy. My GP recommended antidepressants and suggested psychiatric help for my rages. So, I followed his advice and began seeing a psychiatrist.

Besides the emotional turmoil, I was suffering with daily migraines that would begin in the afternoon and continue until I went to sleep at night. In addition to the migraines, I also had insomnia for which I was prescribed sleeping tablets.

Then there were the sore breasts that were so painful at times I couldn't even buckle my seat belt. The litany of complaints continued with severe bloating, frequent urination, extreme fatigue (diagnosed as chronic fatigue), worsening eye sight, dizzy spells that were with me on and off for ten years, reduced sex drive, dry and aging skin, increased blood pressure, food sensitivities, chronic constipation, aches and pains throughout my body, dry and lifeless hair and skin so sensitive that if I was touched it felt raw and exposed. I felt premenstrual all the time. I was once a fit athlete but now my muscle strength had deteriorated to such an extent that I could hardly lift my briefcase.

What added to my despair was discovering that my teeth had lost 50-70 percent of their bone density. All my doctors' warnings that without HRT I would become a victim to the ravages of osteoporosis were proven absurd since my excessive bone loss coincided with the increased use of HRT.

I'm sure that if I wasn't such a strong person I would have certainly attempted suicide. There were times when my life seemed like such a nightmare that I wished I just wouldn't wake up in the morning. The worst part was the fear that my life was careening totally out of my control.

Throughout the years, I made endless visits to doctors... gynecologists, neurologists, ophthalmologists, internists and psychiatrists. I spent thousands of dollars on office visits, tests and medications without benefiting one iota. Not once during all those years, did any doctor ever suggest that HRT could be behind all these symptoms. In fact, I was told that I would have to remain on estrogen for the rest of my life.

From a once healthy, vital, athletic, positive person, I had become devoid of energy, health and self-esteem. Even my once alert and active mind had deserted me. I felt as though I had rapidly arrived at old age. I was convinced that I was dying as all the life energy seemed to be sucked from me. I prayed for a miracle.

The miracle arrived in the form of a friend insisting that I read some information about estrogen dominance, the side-effects of HRT and the benefits of natural progesterone. Since my health felt so delicately balanced on a precipice, I was scared and confused about any kind of change. It took me some time before I was able to gather the courage to try this new avenue.

My first decisive step was to cut my Ogen from 3 tablets to 1 1/2. I literally went cold turkey for six weeks enduring incredible withdrawal symptoms which included an extreme feeling of being disconnected from myself, aches and pains, sadness, sweats, and dizziness to the point of almost passing out. My resolve paid off, however, when after that time my migraines ceased as did my dizziness. I then began to use a transdermal cream of natural progesterone. I know it sounds incredible, but within ten minutes I started to giggle (a rare experience for me at that time) and my mood lifted and I felt as though I had emerged from a fog. After four days my energy began to return and my bloating started to go down.

I also began to see a holistic doctor who was informed about estrogen dominance and natural alternatives. He verified my condition as estrogen dominant. His diagnostic tests showed that my toxicity levels were so high that they were equal to someone who had cancer! It was an understatement to say that my body was a mess! No wonder why I had felt so crazy. I committed to his program of detoxification, dietary changes, nutritional support and natural progesterone cream.

It is now three months since I first began using the cream. My energy increases daily. My anger has disappeared entirely and I'm feeling "up" ninety-five percent of the time. I'm sleeping more soundly now and reducing my sleeping tablets. My mind is clear and sharp and my intuition is flowing again. My dry and itching skin is retuning to its earlier softness. Even the wrinkles are fading! My digestion is improving and I am no longer bloated. My husband and I are living happily together once again and I'm so grateful for all his infinite patience, loyalty and understanding.

All the years I was on HRT were as though I was living a zombie existence and now, at long last, I have finally returned to the land of the living! I now find myself laughing and enjoying life more than I ever did before. There is no doubt in my mind that HRT was the cause of all the symptoms, physically and emotionally, that plagued me during all those years. My anger at being abused by the medical profession has transformed into a burning passion to get the message out to as many women as possible about the dangers, risks as well as safe alternatives to HRT.

I have grown immensely from this intense period of my life. I learned that menopause can be a really positive and empowering change in a woman's life. I now live everyday filled not only with an overflowing gratitude for everything and everyone but with a new and profound appreciation for myself as a woman.

Terri's Story

At 27 years of age, I was experiencing hot flashes and really bad night sweats. In addition I was tired all the time, had insomnia, headaches, aching hands, an aching neck, mild depression and no sex drive. I first noticed these symptoms, especially the hot flashes, four years ago. However, at that time my GP assured me that there was nothing to worry about.

Since my symptoms continued to get worse my GP did another series of tests. This time the tests showed that my estrogen levels were low. He pointed the finger at stress. Since I was working long hours, gruelling hours at a stressful job as a TV producer as well as enjoying a rather active social time, I thought it was all starting to catch up with me. I decided to take time off to take care of myself and did nothing but rest and sleep.

When my symptoms continued, I was referred to an endocrinologist who suggested that I may be going through an early menopause and discussed the possibility of going on to an IVF program and sent me off to do a battery of tests over the next six weeks. I was also immediately taken off the Pill which I had been on continuously since I was fifteen years old (which I now believe was a major contributing factor in my long history of hormonal imbalance).

When all the test results were in, the specialist announced that even though it wasn't exactly known what my problem was, it was decided to prescribe HRT for me anyway and told me to chart my symptoms. I began taking a half of .625 mg. of Ogen. When I asked her about the possible side-effects, she told me not to worry about it and sent me on my way.

After a short time, my hot flashes were reduced but my headaches increased to three time or more a week, I was constantly fatigued and generally felt unwell.

For more than a year I stayed on the HRT. When my hot flashes and night sweats returned, I sought out several other opinions but the answers were all the same. I had early menopause and was told, in fact, to increase the dose of HRT. Within a year I was taking two tablets of .625 mg. Ogen daily.

I was now feeling absolutely terrible. I was unable to work for a year. My motivation was gone as was my self-esteem. I was totally exhausted, continued to have regular headaches, hot flashes, no sex drive and aching neck and hands. I became so depressed that I was further prescribed antidepressants.

By this time, I was really concerned about my ability to have a child so I investigated an IVF program. In order to evaluate my hormone levels, I was told to go off my HRT. When I expressed my concern about going cold turkey, the nurse said I would "just have to handle it."

It was a nightmare. Going cold turkey gave me debilitating migraines. I had intense hot flashes every five minutes and such bad night sweats that I didn't sleep for five nights. I sank deeper into depression assuming that the increase in symptoms meant that my health was deteriorating. I was never warned that the HRT was addictive and that by not taking HRT I could be plunged into instant withdrawals. It never dawned on me that I was a "estrogenaholic".

In the darkest depths of my despair, I chanced upon information explaining the effects of estrogen dominance. I immediately recognized all my symptoms! I sought out a holistic doctor who confirmed my suspicions. I was diagnosed with estrogen dominance. He also said that my liver was damaged due to the toxic effects of the Pill. He immediately began to wean me off of HRT with a natural progesterone cream, changed my diet (eliminating dairy, sugar and wheat while increasing vegetables, fruits and grains) and began a detoxifying program.

After two months on this program, I am now feeling wonderful. My headaches are gone along with my depression. For the first time in over a year I'm excited again with the prospect of going back to work. I have energy in abundance and all my aches and pains have disappeared, My hot flashes and night sweats are almost gone. The most exciting news is that my doctor promises me that my body will be totally rebalanced within a year and that I will be fit and healthy to conceive a child.

I have just turned 29 years old, and I feel like I have finally gotten my life back. I also realize that I was misdiagnosed and misprescribed from the beginning. I was never going through an early menopause. The combination of the Pill and stress certainly triggered my earlier symptoms. I know now that it was the high dose of estrogen in combination with the synthetic progestins in the HRT that really sent my health and emotional well being plummeting into the worst time of my life. I trusted all the experts who really hadn't a clue about what was wrong with me and therefore actually contributed to making the problem much worse.

If I hadn't come across the information about estrogen dominance and found a sympathetic, holistic doctor, I shudder to think what would have happened to me, physically and emotionally. I was certainly heading for big trouble. I'm finally learning to listen to the wisdom of my body and to find the safest and most natural approaches to restore harmony. I have also learned in a very personal way that my health is the most precious thing I have. Without it, nothing else really matters.

Linda's Story

I began using the Pill at the age of seventeen at the insistence of my father. Even though I wasn't sexually active at the time, he, no doubt, thought he was doing the right thing by encouraging me to take preventative measures. I went off the Pill for a year, then back on again for another two years before taking another year's break. I resumed the Pill four years ago at the age of 24 when I entered a committed relationship. During that 'on and off' time I didn't particularly notice any symptoms but then again I was young and wasn't aware of those sorts of things.

Two years ago, I began to notice a number of symptoms that were affecting my body and mind. Symptoms that could be categorized as PMS became progressively more severe. I became very bloated with my stomach protruding out and becoming very hard. There was also excessive fluid retention. My breasts and nipples were becoming so sore and painful that I couldn't stand to get hugged. I also was now getting really intense cramps at the beginning of my period. They would be so severe that all I could do was lie in a fetal position in bed during the first day of my period until they subsided. My periods were becoming heavier and I would have a discharge for several days after they finished. I also discovered noticeable hair growth....those dark, thick kind. They were appearing on different parts of my body —my jaw line, between my breast and even on my big toes! My head hair, however, was falling out. Mentally my thinking was really foggy around ovulation time. I would inevitably make unnecessary mistakes at work at that time.

The long list of symptoms continued. My libido disappeared

'big time'. Floating, sparkling flecks would often appear as though swimming in my field of vision. I have a family history of varicose veins and while on the Pill they appeared and became quite prominent. I experienced excruciating pains in my lower back on the day my period began. I felt like I just wanted to bend my body all the way over backwards to alleviate the pain. There was also the weight gain of more than seven pounds.

What really started to weak havoc with my life, however, were the emotional outbursts. I became extremely critical of everyone and everything, especially myself. I would find myself picking on my partner for the smallest thing which would always wind up in a fight. About two weeks before my period I would transform into the most angry, irrational person. There were times when I could hardly contain the rage and other times when I would fall into a heap and burst into tears for no apparent reason. These symptoms became more extreme with each month. At first I would have these PMS symptoms two weeks out of the month, then three weeks and then it seemed as though I was in a perpetual state of PMS. My life became a living hell. My life was totally out of my control and I felt terrified as though I were completely possessed by unwanted demonic forces.

Throughout those years of physical and emotional pain, my partner's unconditional support and love helped me through the most difficult of times. He was the one who would often recognize that my symptoms were hormonally related. He was usually much more aware of my monthly cyclic changes and their Jeckyl and Hyde effect on me.

I was disappointed, to say the least, that during the entire time I was on the Pill I was never given adequate information from doctors. Although I was once warned of the risk of strokes and blood clots from the Pill, none of its side-effects nor its other potential dangers were ever mentioned. Certainly the Pill was never mentioned at all as a possible cause for my symptoms.

In desperation, I began using a transdermal natural progesterone cream. It took me a little while to really get serious about using it. When I finally committed in the second month to the twice daily application, positive changes began to happen. My breast tenderness stopped completely as did the bloating and fluid retention. I no longer had cramps nor heavy bleeding. The lower back pain disappeared. My thinking became alert again, as though a fog had lifted. And even my libido made its return debut!!! Most incredibly, my emotional life came back into balance. I no longer felt irritable and negative. I began to feel beautiful within myself once again! Instead of lethargically moping around the house with a rather unkempt, grubby appearance, I suddenly was motivated to look after myself and my appearance again. My self-esteem emerged as though awakening from the Pill's spell.

All these changes occurred while I was using the natural progesterone cream even though I was still on the Pill. I also made dietary changes as well as paying more attention to my cyclic wisdom, charting my menstrual cycles and tuning into the moon etc.

As I became more aware of myself as a woman, it became obvious to me that the Pill was no longer appropriate. About four months ago, I decided to stop taking it altogether. I'm still in the process of balancing out my body after it's intense assault from all those years on the synthetic hormones. I'm also eating more healthily, learning to take more time for myself and consulting with a Chinese Herbalist. My physical and emotional health has improved immensely and am aware that I am now walking a path not only of greater hormonal balance but also personal power.

Sally's Story

I went through a comparatively early menopause in my mid-forties. The shock of my mother's unexpected death seemed to trigger my symptoms. Within a very short time I was experiencing night sweats (though no hot flashes) in addition to other medical problems brought on through grief.

At that time I was not seeing a gynecologist and didn't pay much notice to my symptoms. It was only when I went to a woman's clinic for a routine mammogram (I have a family history of breast cancer) that I mentioned my symptoms to an attending doctor.

After a consultation I was put on an HRT with estrogen pills. I was told that I would feel marvellous and 'back to normal' (whatever that is). I tried a number of different brands trying to find one that suited my body. None made me feel well or, in fact, better in any way. In addition I was now bloated and having headaches which I now suspect were exaggerated by the progestin, Primulut.

When I tried to use patches, I discovered I was allergic to the adhesive backing which caused me to break out in water blisters.

I was, therefore, advised to try implants. In addition to a full implant of estrogen, I also was given a 50 percent strength implant of testosterone—the latter supposedly to give energy and impetus to carry on my business life. When I had the first of these, I immediately felt much better very quickly. I had this initial rush of euphoria accompanied with lots of energy and improved sleep . After a couple of weeks, things settled down. The only problem was an increase in fluid retention which seemed to all settle in my buttocks and thighs. I was advised to have a new implant every six months.

However, as the initial benefits began to wear off, I felt like a clock rapidly "winding down". To counteract this problem I decided to put myself onto a timetable of a new implant every four months. There was never a problem about having it done so frequently since no doctor ever questioned my decision nor asked me to have a blood test to determine the level of estrogen in my blood.

It was only at my sister's instigation and insistence that I finally went to see her gynecologist. The doctor insisted on a blood test before she would give me my requested new implant. The results showed that my estrogen level was extremely high. Despite this result, I was desperately needing a "fix".

My doctor refused to give me another implant until my levels had become normal. For the following 18 months I had a monthly blood test to monitor the levels. Each month she refused until she was happy with the results.

Of course, when she refused to give me another implant I was forced to go off "cold turkey". I didn't realize at the time how addictive implants were nor was I prepared for how shocking I would feel. The withdrawal symptoms included extreme fatigue, loss of energy and an accompanying lack of enthusiasm for life. My sleeplessness also returned.

Finally, when my levels were sufficiently reduced, I received another implant. This time it was only estrogen since I was concerned about the testosterone I had been absorbing into my body. What bliss! Within a couple of days, I was on another high!

However, by now I was starting to question where I was going and what was happening to my body. I was really uncomfortable with estrogen's effect on my weight gain which went from 126 lbs. to about 135 lbs. My clothes no longer fit so I gave about half of my wardrobe away. I was tired of people commenting on how much weight I had gained. It was apparent to me that as long as I stayed on the estrogen there was nothing I could do to lose the extra pounds. It became more and more obvious to me that this wasn't what my body wanted.

After being introduced to information about the symptoms and dangers of estrogen excess and its addictive nature, I immediately identified myself as having a dependency on the implants—a little like a heroin junkie. Since I used to be a heavy smoker, I knew how difficult it can be to break an addiction. I was concerned that my addictive tendencies would keep me hooked on my implant.

To cut a long story short, I completely stopped using HRT. Once again I went cold turkey but this time with the help of natural progesterone cream. One year on I feel so much better. My breasts are less sore and less lumpy. My energy level has improved and my weight is getting back to normal. The fluid retention has disappeared and my attitude toward life is once again enthusiastic. I have since been trying out a number of natural progesterone products to find out which one suits me the best.

I have been extremely lucky that through all my problems from the initial symptoms through to the withdrawals some years later, I have had the never ending consideration and love of my husband. Without his support and care, I don't know what would have happened.

Last November, my gynecologists found a lump deep in my left breast—the one that had been "lumpy" on the side for some time. This lump was in the middle of the breast. A breast surgeon scheduled a biopsy a month later. Fortunately for me the lump was benign. It was a condition known as radial scar. In conversation with my surgeon, she commented that she was seeing more and more women with breast lumps of various kinds in the years since HRT had become popular.

She said that since she was approaching her menopausal years, she decided never to take HRT because of its implication with an increased risk of breast cancer.

I have personally persuaded many women, both friends and acquaintances, to stop using HRT and to consider a more natural approach such as including soy products in their diet and using natural progesterone cream. I'm once again like the zealous reformed smoker I was many years ago! Since giving up HRT my body is on the mend. I now find myself wanting to inform as many women as possible about the safe and natural alternatives to HRT so they can potentially avoid serious health problems in the future.

PART THREE

The Feminine Path to Power

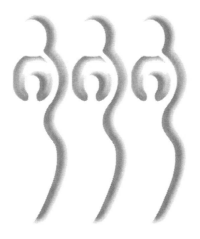

Chapter 1

Looking into the Crystal Ball

Four hundred years ago, Nostradamus, perhaps the most famous of all visionaries, foresaw that the end of this millennium would usher in an unprecedented period of history when the influence of the feminine would transform all of society. His powerful predictions announced the end of the patriarchal order which has so dominated the course of history for the past five thousand years. This predicted ascendancy of the feminine will be responsible for not only initiating a massive experience of human renewal but also a completely new vision of how all of life can be an expression of harmony.

Included in his prophecies was the prediction that medical science would find ways of healing the body through formerly misunderstood natural cycles. He went on to reveal how the balance of hormones in a woman connects her with and aligns her to the earth's rhythms. Returning to the understanding of a woman's cyclic nature will restore the magic of the feminine and the wisdom of her instinctual nature. Nostradamus believed that only by such a transformation could humanity's survival be assured.

So, as we arrive at that predicted point in time, a massive awakening of women is required to fulfil the promise of Nostradamus' inspirational vision. Never before in history have so many millions of women sacrificed their hormonal balance, thus themselves, into the embrace of medical science. Besides creating devastating health problems which are only now coming to light, synthetic hormones have so altered a woman's natural rhythms that her powerful connection to her inner sense of Self has been seriously compromised.

What would it be like to know that in the deepest depths of your being as a woman, every part of your anatomy and each process of your female body contained ancient wisdom, a wellspring of creativity and unfathomable power?

Since entering a new millennium, it appears that women are also welcoming a new sense of self. The essential nature of a woman is cyclical, expressed by her monthly flow of changing hormones, energies and emotions. Life is about recurring cycles. It is expressed in the changing rhythms of the moon and the seasons. It is also found in the cosmic cycles described by the ancient sciences of astrology and numerology. The return of the feminine and women's awakening to a deeper appreciation of themselves is part of a greater cycle.

Chapter 2

Forgotten History

Extensive archeological research has now verified that beginning approximately 38,000 years ago humanity worshipped the feminine principle personified in the symbolism of the Goddess.

From Old Europe through Greece, Egypt, the Near East, India and the Far East, the Great Goddess was perceived as an organizing principle of the universe who embodied all the forces of life, death and rebirth within her figure. Her dominion encompassed not only the human world but also the plant and animal realms, earth and heaven and the seasonal and sky cycles. The Goddess was the embodiment of the life force that animated all of existence.

The Goddess religions embraced the constant and periodic renewal of life in which death was not separate from life. This religion displayed a deep respect for the natural cycles of women. In the societies where she was worshipped, women held exalted roles as priestesses, leaders, healers, midwives and diviners. These cultures held a deep reverence for the earth as the giver of life. The female form represented the embodiment of the power of nature.

Noting the correlation of the twenty nine days for the moon cycle with the twenty nine days of women's menstrual cycles, the ancients surmised the moon must be feminine. The rhythm of the moon, whose phases resonated to women's menstrual cycles, held a special place in the myths, religion and symbols of the Goddess. The Goddess teachings held that death was but the precursor to rebirth and that sex could be used not only for procreation but also for ecstasy, healing, regeneration and spiritual illumination.

Archeological remains from these cultures show no evidence of fortifications, weapons or violent deaths from warring. For tens of thousands of years these Goddess-oriented cultures lived in peace and harmony with equality between the sexes. The art, artifacts and earliest writings of these peoples documented that they were peaceful agriculturists, living harmoniously in matrilineal partnership societies.

The Feminine is Forgotten

All this began to change about five thousand years ago when warring tribes from northern Europe and central Asia descended into western Europe, the Near East and India. They invaded, conquered and destroyed the indigenous Goddess cultures.

It was a violent time when the patriarchal solar Gods overthrew the Mother Goddess. Women were stripped of their positions of political authority and their decision making powers as leaders. They were deprived of their spiritual authority as priestesses. Banned from functioning in their professional and healing capacities, they were progressively disempowered from expressing their sexuality, intelligence and self-sufficiency.

The emergence of the major world religions usurped the power of the feminine declaring that which once was sacred to be taboo. The Inquisition and witch hunts of the Middle Ages was a determined effort by the Church and State to eliminate the last vestiges of the influence and power of the Goddess. It is estimated that nine million women were systematically murdered during a three hundred year period.

The Patriarchy now ruled supreme. Inherent in this culture was blind obedience to the male principle embodied by the father. It was based on the supremacy of the intellect, rigid rules, violence, control over others and the environment, efficiency and suppression of spontaneity and emotions. Women were relegated to second class citizens and considered the property of men. Women and all womanly functions were denigrated, defiled and became synonymous with evil.

Western civilization, embodying the legacy of patriarchy, has exalted all things male. It demands that women ignore or turn away from their hopes and dreams in deference to men and the demands of their families. The systematic stifling of the need for self-expression and self-actualization causes women enormous emotional pain. To stay out of touch with that pain, women have commonly used addictive substances and developed dysfunctional behaviors that have resulted in an endless cycle of abuse towards themselves, their bodies and others.

The five thousand year old patriarchal system is encoded within the very psyche of women. It has been passed down from generation to generation of women. It shapes their behaviors, attitudes and the very health of their bodies. It is the force that drives women to exhaustion, unable to stop long enough to attend to their own needs. It creates their obsession with a body that is never perfect enough. It is why women seek external authority to tell them how to live their own lives. It ensures that women remain economically, politically and spiritually helpless and dependent.

It is also the reason why women are filled with shame, disgust and guilt towards their bodies and normal female functions. It taunts them by calling menstruation 'the curse'. It is behind the millions of women who suffer each month with PMS—a symptom of their rejection of their feminine self.

It contributes to almost 50 percent of western women who have hysterectomies. It is why 60 percent of women experience painful periods each month—the majority of whom suffer in silence.

The Awakening

The re-emergence of the Feminine now stirring within the

hearts of women is the call to reclaim all that has been kept hidden from them. Reclaiming this wisdom begins with honoring the cyclic nature of women. Women are lunar in nature. Just as the moon continues to cycle through its changes each month, so, too, do women. The menstrual cycle is the most basic cycle women have. The flow of blood is a woman's connection to the archetypal feminine. In many cultures the menstrual cycle was viewed as sacred because it reconnects a woman with the creative principles of the universe.

The menstrual cycle governs not only the flow of fluids, but also information and creativity. The ebb and flow of dreams, intuition and hormones associated with different parts of the cycle offer women a profound opportunity to deepen their connection to their inner knowing.

Information is received and processed differently during each phase of the cycle. Brooke Medicine Eagle, Native American teacher and author affirms, "there is a spiritual power and beauty that builds in a woman who honors that part of herself. That's how women in native cultures got to be so wise."

Each month a woman recapitulates the phases of creation, nourishment, death and regeneration. From the first day of menstruation until ovulation is the follicular phase. During this time, her power can be used to conceive artistic and intellectual offspring as well as actual biological children.

It is the time when women are most outgoing and attractive to men (volatile hormones are secreted) and it culminates at the time of the full moon.

If pregnancy does not occur, the second half of the cycle is known as the luteal phase—from ovulation until the onset of menstruation. This is the time when there is a desire to retreat from outer activity to a more reflective mode. This inner space nurtures the opportunity to develop or give birth to something that comes from deep within. Menstruation correlates to the dark phase of the moon.

At this time women are most in tune with their inner knowing and understanding of what isn't working in their lives. Premenstrually, the 'veil between the worlds' of the seen and unseen, the conscious and the unconscious, is much thinner. It is when intuitive wisdom is the strongest and dreams most revealing. There is access to parts of the often unconscious self that are less available at all other times of the month. At this time women are able to connect to their magic—their ability to change things for the better because they are most sensitive to their inner selves.

In the Native American tradition, menstruating women would retire together to the moon lodge. This was a time for renewal and visioning. The women emerged afterward inspired and inspiring to others. Perhaps the majority of PMS cases would disappear if every modern woman gave herself permission to retreat from her duties for three or four days each month to her own personal 'moon lodge'.

Lunar Consciousness

The masculine world is based upon solar consciousness—the linear, rational, predictable rhythm of life. Lunar consciousness, however, requires listening and responding to the ever-changing inner impulses of instinctual wisdom. If a woman does not understand the need for slowing down and honoring the more introspective energy during the luteal phase, then intuitive information is unable to be received. This ignored information may then manifest as PMS or menopausal madness, in the same way that ignored feelings and bodily symptoms often result in disease. To the extent that women are out of touch with the hidden parts of themselves, they will suffer premenstrually and menopausally.

If a woman is in attunement with her menstrual wisdom, then each month she will be renewed and cleansed—physically, emotionally and spiritually. It was not necessary for Native American women to participate in the sweat lodge ceremony—a male ritual for purification—because it was understood that she was purified each month. Honoring such natural cycles can transform Premenstrual Syndrome into Premenstrual Strength.

The Truth About Menopause

If a woman is in harmony with her physical self as well as her deeper emotional and spiritual self, she is then prepared to enter the final initiation of her sacred woman's power—menopause.

In the patriarchal system, menopause has been made into the most dreaded and terrifying inevitability. Unlike men, who gain esteem and power as they age, menopausal women are perceived as losing their attractiveness and sexuality—literally and figuratively 'drying up'. How truly threatening this time is to women if their entire sense of worth is connected with being attractive to men. Menopause is also associated with loss of health, memory, independence, usefulness and creativity. In fact, most of the symptoms attributed to menopause are really the result of a stressful life-style which has created a huge imbalance in a woman's life and body.

The ancient Goddess cultures and many of today's indigenous cultures, knew the truth about menopause. It was the fullest blossoming of a woman's power, wisdom and creativity. Menopause was the initiation into the Wise Woman stage of life. In Native American tradition, it was only upon entering menopause that women were ready to become the Medicine Women and Shamans of their tribes. It was a position of the utmost respect.

For women to fulfil their potential during this second half of their lives, many myths must be shed. The conventional medical mind-set is that menopause is a deficiency disease not a natural process. It is believed to be a time when the ovaries dry up. Just as women's bodies have become pathologized and medicalized by the patriarchal, addictive system, so too has every function unique to women, menopause included.

As we have already explored, the ovaries go through changes during menopause, reducing estrogen and progesterone levels and altering their functions to produce other hormones. By no means do they shrivel up and cease functioning, as popular belief has it. In addition, other body sites such as the adrenal glands, skin, muscle, brain, pineal gland, hair follicles and body fat, are capable of making these essential hormones. Nature assists the female body to make healthy adjustments, in hormonal balance after menopause, providing a woman has taken good care of herself during the perimenopausal years.

In a most enlightening book called *Creative Menopause*, Farida Sharan states, "Menopause is a movement upwards. When we come into our forties and fifties, the tide of procreative sexuality and outward energies begins to shift inward and upward. As our ovaries release our last eggs and our hormones change, the challenge and the opportunity to open our higher centers of consciousness becomes a reality we face every day, either consciously or unconsciously. If we cling to what is already passing away, we get stuck. Disease patterns and mental and emotional imbalances are out of our refusal to move and change. But if we cooperate consciously with the process, the treasures that lie ahead will be greater than exploring the new world or space frontiers. Our unborn, uncharted being awaits to prepare us for our next level of emergence in the life of spirit."

She goes on to say, "When we complete menopause we move beyond the alternating cyclic nature and become like a direct current, charged and focused with the ability to speak and act truth and to express directly who we are through our inner vision. Certainly there is a tremendous shift of energy which is both liberating and powerful. We need to cooperate fully with this process to make the most of this creative opportunity.

As attention shifts to the inner world, away from the personal into the universal, we learn to enjoy what is being given in our elder years and we do not want to waste time in fear and negativity by longing for what has already passed away."

Menopausal women have the opportunity to enter into a time of life fully empowered in their wisdom and creativity. It is the beginning of a whole new cycle of freedom and inner knowing.

The feminine path to power requires a woman to reclaim her own authority over her life—her needs, her rhythms and her body—and to trust her own instinctual nature once again. It's about realizing that she is not separate from nature but rather an expression of nature. Physical or emotional problems are expressions of disharmony. They are the messengers that let her know she is out of balance with some aspect of her life.

Self-healing requires personal disarmament, refusing to be at war any longer with a part of your body that's trying to tell you something. As women awaken, they will no longer need to deny or violate themselves in any way.

Shedding all the internalized messages of blame, self-doubt and self-hatred that are encoded within the cells frees each woman to attune to her inner guidance. Then she will always know when to be active and when to be quiet; when to care for others and when to care for self; when she is following her instinctual wisdom and when she is being directed by old conditioning. Therein lies her true source of power.

Like emerging from a long, deep period of hibernation, women all over the world are awakening to a power within themselves that has laid dormant for so very long. Feminine power is not the same as male power. Feminine power emanates directly from a woman's wholeness. Only by reclaiming the banished sacred Feminine Self can women truly realize their deepest hopes and dreams for themselves, their families and Mother Earth.

Creating Sacred Feminine Power

The following are suggestions to support the blossoming of Women's Wisdom.

1. Journal—keep a daily account of your inner most thoughts and feelings.

2. Become aware of the moon and all her phases. Bask in the moonlight. Honor the moon as the archetype of the feminine. It has been shown that the light of the full

moon increases levels of follicle stimulating hormone (FSH) via the hypothalamus and pituitary glands.

3. Take time either by yourself or with friends to have a full moon meditation.

4. Listen to your Menstrual Wisdom. When entering into the luteal stage, listen to your body. Take quiet time for yourself. Rest if you feel tired. Be daring and take a nap during the day! Allow your feelings to be expressed.

5. Keep a dream book to record your dreams and inner visions. Be especially aware of your dreams right before your period.

6. Buy a moon calendar to keep track of the moon's cycles each month.

7. Write into your diary when you will be experiencing your menstrual cycles.

8. Spend time alone with nature. Become aware of her rhythms and cycles, recognizing that you share her rhythms.

Chapter 3

Women's Power and Women's Health Choices

The challenge of the modern woman is to be able to face the dragons of modern medicine, fully empowered, intuitive instincts intact and with the ability to say "No" if necessary. She also needs adequate self-esteem to set limits, to ask for what she wants and needs and the courage to seek and find all the appropriate guidance and support for her health needs.

The origins of disease are many—heredity, constitutional weaknesses, aging factors, life-style along with spiritual, mental and emotional causes. Even though there are times when we don't know why our body is giving us problems, we need to be open to exploring the ways that we have contributed to this "dis-ease" within ourselves. Have we been worrying excessively, not eating properly, or perhaps pushing ourselves to expend energy we don't have?

Whenever some illness is occurring, we must take some time and listen for the inner messages to discover what our body is trying to tell us. Instead of expecting doctors to be solely responsible for fixing us up, we need to learn to participate equally in our own healing process. While we can certainly appreciate modern medical skills and give thanks that they are available should we ever need them, we must not become a passive bystander regarding the needs of our own body. It is imperative that we become directly and therapeutically involved in our healing process—after all, who's body is it, anyway?

We can also learn how to adjust our daily lives, eliminating any habit that does not support our total well-being. We are now being asked to take a higher level of responsibility for our own lives.

Modern medicine developed out of mechanistic and scientific thinking that did not consider the important effects of the mind, emotions and spirit on our physical condition. This system disregards the whole person and focuses entirely on the physical. Modern medicine also regards the body as a machine and believes that when a part of the machine fails, the efficient treatment is to fix the part or replace it. True healing, which takes into account all aspects of a person's life, is rarely offered.

Orthodox medicine, based on this patriarchal, scientific paradigm, does not respect anything that cannot be logically and rationally seen, measured or proven. Much of life and death is invisible and immeasurable, as are feelings, thoughts and spiritual realities. The definable, measurable realities are only a small part of our life experience.

A New Understanding of the Mind/Body

Dr. Deepak Chopra, a pioneer of Mind/Body Medicine and author of the best selling book *Quantum Healing*, has said that our bodies are more like a flowing river rather than a sculpture frozen in time. Every thought, every emotion, every perception is directly and instantaneously affecting our bodies— either in the direction of healing or in the direction of disease.

We need to respect doctors and surgeons for their devoted years of study, their sacrifices and their remarkable skills. While this respect should not be eroded, neither should we regard them as the source of absolute control and authority over our bodies and our lives. We have the right to question or even refuse their suggestions for treatment. We must be fully informed and responsible for the decisions we make, the medicines we accept and whatever else we allow to be done to us. We do not have to offer ourselves up helplessly to the dictates of modern medicine.

We can cooperate fully and intelligently with the best of whatever is being offered medically and freely choose to explore other educational, therapeutic, natural, spiritual and complementary healing options.

The medical system is there to serve us. When we interact with doctors and the medical system, we must also be willing to challenge them to expand and grow. We must demand communication and respect. We must educate ourselves not only about our bodies but also the many psychological and spiritual changes that occur during a woman's life. As we discover the courage to seek out those who can help us, we must overcome feelings of fear, helplessness and despair. Whatever needs are not being provided for outside ourselves, we must now turn within, discovering the abundant strength and wisdom of our own inner resources.

When a menopausal woman seeks advice from her doctor for her health problems, the physical aspect of the menopausal symptoms usually becomes the focus. Menopause is often inaccurately blamed for other life-style, aging and disease symptoms. Generally a doctor is ill-equipped to understand and assist her with the spiritual unfolding and emotional transformation that is taking place. Everything is blamed on her hormones and the menopause. She is told that her ovaries are failing and the womb is often seen as irrelevant.

But menopause is not just a physical change, it is one of the most important spiritual stages in our life—an initiation into the blossoming of our Woman's Wisdom. Unfortunately, most women arrive at the time of menopause exhausted—physically, emotionally and mentally—from the relationship, family and work responsibilities that have consumed their attention for so many years of their lives. Since mid-life is a time of harvest, problems and issues that in the past have been ignored now surface demanding resolution. Life is demanding that we become the priority of our lives. Somehow we must find the time and energy to give to ourselves as we move through this passage. However much we have given of ourselves—to our loved ones, our work and our world—now is the time to fully give to ourselves. Such is the path to a woman's true power.

Women travel through many stages and initiations in their lives—from the onset of menstruation into motherhood and then menopause. With each stage, we must learn to make the necessary changes and adjustments that correspond to that time of life—with diet and lifestyle, emotional and creative expression and spiritual needs. Each stage is important and bestows upon us special gifts as we garner our learnings and wisdom throughout life.

Certainly women have it well within their own power not only to find safe, natural and effective ways to balance and heal themselves but to live long, full lives while preserving their vitality, youthfulness and health. Women deserve the right to appreciate themselves and their bodies through all the stages of life. As women find the way to return to a greater balance within themselves, they will profoundly know the truth of their immense contribution to Life.

PART FOUR

Returning to Balance

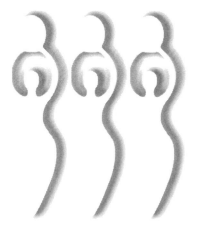

Chapter 1

Walking the Middle Path

Buddha's greatest advice to the seekers of enlightenment was to walk the Middle Path. The Middle Path is about living in harmony and balance within ourselves. Finding balance is like walking a tight rope—each step along the wire requires rebalancing. Balance is a dynamic process; it changes with the days, the seasons, the years. To be so sensitive to oneself and one's needs that adjustments are made easily and quickly seems to be the key to living happily and peacefully. Welcoming change is an essential ingredient of the Middle Path. Without the willingness to change, the tight rope walker would quickly plunge to the ground.

Living life so that we may savor the many experiences along the way is an art. Life reveals its many secrets and wisdoms as we live it. The guides along this journey are our intuition, natural instincts and inner wisdom. They are the true jewels that we all possess. What is truly precious, however, may take a lifetime to discover.

To attain peace of mind it is essential to be committed to living in balance with oneself. Illness, emotional pain, unhappiness and confusion are merely symptoms of disharmony—they are the 'taps on our shoulders' attempting to tell us that we are out of sync with our Self in some way.

Restoring hormonal balance for a woman requires her to bring all aspects of her life into greater harmony and alignment. It is not just about taking some medication or treatment, no matter how natural. In every moment a woman's body is expressing her innermost needs. How adept she is at responding will reflect in her overall physical, emotional and mental well-being. There are times when we may fool ourselves. There are times when we can fool others. But we can never fool our body. It is the most sensitive barometer of our inner world.

A healthy plant has many requirements—the right amount of sun, correct temperature, adequate water, proper nutrients and careful weeding. All these factors are equally necessary for the plant's growth. We, too, have many requirements to sustain our growth. Balance is effortlessly attained if we honor and implement our essential ingredients for growth.

The following are suggestions for returning to balance. Some are absolutely essential while others fall into the category of optional choices. There are many ways to rebalance and each woman must find the way that is most appropriate and useful to her. Listen to your inner wisdom to find your way and have the courage to follow it.

Chapter 2

Food is Medicine

Proper understanding of diet is essential not only to a maintain a healthy body, but also for balanced emotions and an alert mind. The average Western diet is hopelessly inadequate, out-of-balance and toxic.

Food is medicine for our body. Whatever we eat is either adding to our health or detracting from it. There is no middle ground. Learning the basic guidelines for eating is an obvious and necessary step for regaining balance.

Many excellent books abound that teach nutrition, so I will leave that to them. The following are some fundamental guidelines about what foods to include more often in your diet and what foods are best to reduce or avoid altogether. Scientific studies show that a mostly vegetarian, low-fat, whole food diet is preventative medicine at its finest. Eating organic food—vegetables, fruits, seeds, grains and meats—is becoming a necessity due to mounting evidence of the long-term harm herbicides, pesticides and other xeno-estrogens are doing to our health.

There is some new information about what foods are good for women, so that will be the focus in this section. Lissa De Angelis and Molly Siple, two nutritional counsellors, have co-authored an excellent cookbook book called *Recipes for Change* to assist women to return to hormonal balance through food. I have included their most up-to-date findings which include new nutritional stars such as bioflavonoids, boron, phytohormones and essential fatty acids.

These nutrients, which are found in countless foods, play numerous roles in supporting a woman's body during its many changes.

Bioflavonoids

This group of compounds (which includes citron, hesperidin, rutin and flavanones) has a structure and chemical activity similar to estrogen. By mimicking and modulating estrogen fluctuations, the presence of bioflavonoids in the body has been shown to control hot flashes and the psychological symptoms of menopause including anxiety, irritability and mood swings. Bioflavonoids lessen heavy menstrual bleeding in premenopause, strengthen capillary walls and help to keep the skin healthy and supple. Some of the foods that contain bioflavonoids include green peppers, cherries, buckwheat, rose hips and, especially, citrus, which contains the complete bioflavonoid complex. Bioflavonoids are not destroyed by cooking but remain stable.

Boron

Throughout your life sufficient boron is needed for metabolizing calcium as well as for maintaining motor skills and mental alertness. Two large apples, a cup of broccoli florets or a handful of nuts supplies 1 mg. of boron, a good start for the 1 to 3 mgs of boron per day required for good health. Some other boron-containing foods include millet, buckwheat, whole oats and barley, soybeans, lentils, spinach, potatoes, parsley, beets, green peas, cabbage, asparagus, pears, peaches, grapes, raisins, rockmelons, lemons, bananas, almonds, hazelnuts, walnuts, flax seeds and shrimp. Interestingly, a recent study of women on estrogen replacement therapy seems to indicate that boron can mimic and enhance the action of supplemental estrogen.

Phytohormones

Sometimes called phytoestrogens, phytohormones are

substances found in plant foods that affect your hormone status. They are present in dozens of foods that we commonly eat and these foods have been shown to have an effect on the hormonal balance of the body. Phytohormone potencies are considerably weaker than the estrogen that is produced in your ovaries, called estradiol. Although many of these plant hormones are 1/400th to 1/100,000th the potency of estradiol, they can mimic and modulate estrogens and can help stabilize hormone fluctuations. Some of the phytohormone foods are brown rice, beans, flax seeds, radishes, tofu, pomegranates, rhubarb, potatoes, fennel and green tea. Vegetarian women can have phytohormone levels one hundred times greater than women eating a typical western diet.

Consuming foods rich in phytohormones may also lower your risk of heart disease and breast cancer. Japanese women eating a traditional diet have fewer incidences of hot flashes and lower rates of breast cancer. Scientists have suggested that the consumption of soybeans and soy products like tofu, which are high in phytohormones, is part of the reason. However, the traditional Japanese diet is also low in processed and refined foods and high in mineral-rich seaweed and fresh fish oils— all of which are important factors. It is interesting to note that when Japanese women eat a more western diet, the incidence of heart disease and cancer increases.

Essential Fatty Acids

Essential fatty acids make up the components of many organs and tissues. They bring oxygen to our tissues, help prevent premenstrual symptoms, improve the condition of hair, nails and skin and help prevent all major degenerative diseases, including heart disease and cancer. They are essential for good health throughout life.

There are two families of essential fatty acids, called omega-6 and omega-3. We need about twice as much omega-6 as omega-3. However, most of us are already getting so much omega-6 that we need to seriously boost our consumption of omega-3. Some of the foods high in omega-3 are walnuts, flax seed oil, dark green leafy vegetables and fish. The average healthy adult requires 4 teaspoons of essential oils per day, but a woman in menopause, especially with dry skin, hair and vaginal tissue, may need to 2 or 3 tablespoons per day before her symptoms disappear.

Chapter 3

Foods to Avoid

Refined Sugar

Refined sugars (cane and beet sugar, brown sugar, corn syrup and any word that ends in 'ose', i.e., dextrose) are completely devoid of vitamins, minerals and fiber and have no nutritive value. They stress your body and actually deplete it of vitamins and minerals. Refined sugar can lead to calcium loss and contributes to weight gain, diabetes, tooth and gum disorders, nervous disorders, low blood sugar and fatigue.

Caffeine

Caffeine quickens respiration, increases blood pressure, stimulates the kidneys, excites brain function and temporarily alleviates fatigue and depression. It can create vitamin and mineral deficiencies, prevent iron absorption, irritate the stomach lining, aggravate the heart and arteries and increase nervous symptoms. Caffeine is found in coffee, black teas, chocolate and in many sodas. Coffee is a diuretic. It has few nutrients and stimulates excess excretion of urine along with the vitamins and minerals urine contains.

Processed Oils

Most cooking oils are refined which means that they have

had the flavorful elements, smells and natural colors removed. Corn, canola and safflower oils are all refined. Refined oils contain toxic substances and should be avoided. Hydrogenated fats, such as shortening and margarine, are strongly linked to heart disease and cancer. The beneficial oils are extra-virgin olive oil, flax seed oil, unrefined sesame oil, coconut butter and unsalted butter. Ideally, oils should be organically produced and cold-pressed. Always keep oils refrigerated or they will go rancid.

Refined Flours and Grains

The most nutritional part of the grain (the germ and bran) is removed when processed, leaving the part we buy highly devoid of vitamins, minerals, fiber and essential fatty acids. All whole grains are correctly called complex carbohydrates consisting of the bran, germ and endosperm. Whole grains include whole wheat, brown rice, buckwheat, millet, cornmeal, oatmeal and whole grain pastas. Whenever possible choose products made with whole grains.

Dairy Products

Dairy products are best avoided completely. Contrary to all the dairy industry advertising, it is one of the worst foods a woman can eat. Consumption of dairy products increases symptoms of PMS such as swelling, cramping and breast tenderness. After abstaining from all dairy products (a moderate amount of unsalted butter is acceptable since it is primarily a fat containing very little milk solids or protein) many women have reported shrinking or disappearance of fibroids, less menstrual bleeding and for fewer days, reduced endometriosis pain, improved allergies and sinusitis and lessening of recurrent vaginitis.

Dairy products also contain many added hormones and residues of antibiotics. Dairy foods are a protein. Excessive protein leaches calcium from the bone in order to neutralize the more acidic environment that the proteins create. Therefore dairy products contribute to bone loss!

It is no coincidence that the countries with the highest rates of osteoporosis—the United States, Great Britain and Sweden—are also the countries with the highest dairy consumption.

A Word About Vitamins

It is currently estimated that less than 9 percent of the population eats an adequate amount of vegetables and fruits to maintain high levels of vitamins and minerals in our bodies. Many women throughout their lives are missing vital nutrients. No wonder ill health is so common. While vitamin and mineral tablets are a useful way of supplementing nutrients, they must be taken in conjunction with nutrient-rich food. Together with these foods, supplements can build and fuel a depleted body. Taking supplements without accompanying food is like giving water to a flowerpot that has no plant. Be sure to get proper nutritional advice when choosing vitamins. Just remember, popping vitamin pills will never replace wholesome nutrition.

Chapter 4

Precious Water

When it comes to rebalancing the body, one of the most crucial ingredients is generally overlooked—and that is the most precious, life-giving element on this planet, water! Did you know that water is necessary for optimum brain function, digestion, absorption of nutrients, circulation, hormonal management and all biochemical processes in each of your cells? It is excellent for healthy, clear, soft skin. Scientific research has shown that the better the water management in a cell, the more efficiently proteins, enzymes, hormones and other biochemical elements are able to function. Dehydration can create an imbalance of minerals which will disrupt hormone balance.

So important is the need for proper hydration that the newsletter, *Health Alert*, reported recently, "When it comes to disease like heart, kidney or stomach disease, allergies, asthma, arthritis and skin disease, your state of hydration (water balance) may be the single most important factor in your recovery or even your survival."

Of particular and critical interest to women is the role of chronic dehydration in the development of breast cancer. In his book, *Your Body's Many Cries for Water*, Dr. Batmanchelidj says that the stress that dehydration creates "will increase the secretion of a hormone called prolactin which can at times cause the breast to transform into cancerous tissue. Also, the dehydration would alter the balance of amino acids and allow more DNA errors during cell division."

Dr. Batmanchelidj goes on to say that, "The breast is a water-secreting organ...Whether you are having a child or not makes no difference. The breast must be ready to fulfill its pre-destined role...If a woman already has breast cancer, drinking plenty of water would assist with any therapy by flushing out the toxins. If you do not have breast cancer or want to prevent a metastasis from occurring, it is urgent that you drink enough water. If you don't, your breast may suffer horribly because of its unique role in supplying fluids."

A serious problem these days is a chronic state of dehydration in women. When thirsty it is common to drink coffee, tea, fruit juices, sodas and energy drinks. Unfortunately these drinks do not hydrate the body but rather contribute to dehydration. Only pure water will do! Tap water is generally so polluted with chemical concoctions that it is also dehydrating. Either filtered water or bottled water is the better choice. Generally a woman needs about 1-1.5 liters per day—whether she is thirsty or not!

Hydration is the body's ability to absorb and manage water effectively. Hydration is one of the keys to more energy and improved immunity. It is not how much water you drink but rather how well hydrated your body is. The stresses of daily living—pollution, emotional and physical stress, or inadequate nutrition—can all compromise your body's water balancing mechanism. Simply drinking more water is not always the answer. Just as when water is poured onto a really dried up potted plant and most of it runs right out the bottom, even though you may be drinking lots of water, it too may be pouring right out of you without hydrating your body. The key is getting the body to absorb the water efficiently.

A great way to improve hydration is to drink water regularly throughout the day, especially if you can drink several glasses made with 10-20 percent of organic apple juice. The sugar of the diluted apple juice enhances hydration.

Chapter 5

The Breath of Life

Breathing, like proper water intake, is so often overlooked in our quest for greater balance in our lives. Yet proper breathing is a vital key for assisting longevity, creating balanced hormonal production, increasing energy and reducing stress. It also optimizes athletic performance, enhances concentration and increases confidence. Proper breathing returns our body to balance—physically, emotionally, mentally and spiritually. Filling our body with oxygen is filling it with Life Force. No wonder that breathing has been an intrinsic part of all the ancient wisdoms throughout history.

The key to receiving the healing benefits from the breath is to breathe properly—the way we were designed to breathe. While most people tend to breathe rapidly and only in their upper chest while raising their shoulders as they inhale deeply this, in fact, is known as futile breathing. It is a disastrous breathing style!

Dr. Saul Hendler, a respected medical doctor, comments in his book, *The Oxygen Breakthrough—30 Days to an Illness-free Life*, that futile breathing can cause cardiac symptoms, angina, respiratory symptoms, gastrointestinal distress, anxiety, panic, depression, headache, dizziness, seizures, increased susceptibility to infection and other immune dysfunctions and sleep disturbances. In addition, futile breathing contributes to confused thinking and emotional upset.

A recent article published in the *American Journal of Obstetrics and Gynecology* (167; 436-7) reported that slow, deep breathing reduced the incidence of hot flashes by 50 percent in a group of women who were not on hormone replacement therapy.

Receiving the optimum benefit from the breath, which is really the way nature designed us to breathe, requires drawing the inhaled air all the way down into the very bottom of the lungs so that the diaphragm expands. It's as though the breath were sinking all the way down and then gradually inflating the rest of the lungs. You have taken a correct breath when you are able to fill your lungs fully without lifting your shoulders! The inhale is the more active part of the breath and the exhale is very gentle and relaxed.

I teach this simple breathing technique in my psychotherapy practice with the most profound results. My clients experience feelings of profound peace, mental clarity, emotional balance, an expanded awareness, inner realizations, increased energy and relief from a wide variety of physical problems including hormonal imbalance. I recommend practicing the following breathing exercise for just twenty breaths, twice a day.

The Healing Breath

1. Sitting or lying comfortably, place your hands on your stomach (abdomen).

2. Inhale slowly and deeply through your nose, letting your abdomen expand as though you were filling up the bottom part of a balloon.

3. Allow the breath to first be drawn into the lower lungs, then gradually allow it to fill the upper lungs as well.

4. Relax and gently exhale.

5. Guide the breath into a circular rhythm so that the breath can flow easily from the inhale to the exhale without pausing or stopping.

6. As you feel greater relaxation in your body, allow the inhale to gently expand, taking in fuller breaths.

Chapter 6

Use It or Lose It

Nature designed the body to move. Exercise is an important and essential ingredient for physical and emotional health. It not only tones up your muscles but works on your whole anatomy. It works in conjunction with your metabolism for the better handling of nutrients. In fact, exercise added to nutrients upgrades their effectiveness and efficiency. According to one study, women of childbearing age who exercised four or more hours per week halved their risk of breast cancer before menopause.

Regular exercise will also decrease your risk of heart disease by raising the level of good HDL and lowering bad LDL. It is not surprising that sedentary women are three times more likely to die of heart attacks than women who exercise regularly. You can reduce your risk of dying from a heart attack by 50 percent if you tend to be at risk for heart disease. (By the way, this is the same figure that's been used for Premarin!) Exercise is also directly linked to your hormonal health which is why hot flashes can be reduced by a regular exercise program.

Exercise is beneficial at whatever age you begin. Dr. Deepak Chopra relates a study in his book *Ageless Body, Ageless Wisdom* conducted by gerontologists at Tufts University. They visited a nursing home where they selected a group of the most frail residents and put them on a weight-training regimen. Within eight weeks wasted muscles had come back by 300 percent, coordination and balance improved and overall a sense of active life returned. What makes this accomplishment truly wondrous, however, is that the youngest subject in the group was 87 and the oldest 96!

The real trick to exercise is to like what you do. If the kind of exercise you're doing is more like duty or drudgery, then the benefits won't be as great if you found something that was thoroughly enjoyable. For me, roller blading is an absolute delight. I can happily cruise along on my blades for hours at a time. The time I'm getting my aerobic exercise also fills me with a great sense of pleasure. So, choose your exercise with enjoyment in mind!

To strengthen your bones, some form of weight bearing exercise must be included in your program. Walking uphills, bicycling in low gear, weight training, climbing steps or doing a step machine are all examples providing bone strengthening benefits.

Researchers in St. Louis found that in less than 22 months women who exercised at least three times a week increased their bone density 5.2 percent while sedentary women actually lost 1.2 percent. A recently reported randomized controlled study from Canada found that subjects who exercised for 60 minutes three times a week for a year stabilized their bone mass, improved their cardiovascular endurance and had a better overall sense of well-being than those in the control group.

Chapter 7

Meditation—Moving Inwards

While meditation may conjure up images of exotic, esoteric techniques, it is, in fact, simply learning to settle one's thoughts and to be fully focused in the moment. It offers a time for inner contemplation. There are many ways to attain that centering. Some can be learned through various techniques taught at meditation/relaxation centers or from audio or video tapes. It is also possible to meditate as one listens to favorite music or while just strolling along the beach or in a park. Whatever your preferred way may be, taking time to meditate has clearly been shown to produce marvellous benefits both for one's physical health as well as emotional and spiritual well-being. Besides eliminating the harmful effects of stress, it enables you to tap into your creative energy and even reverse the aging process!

To receive meditation's many rewards, it is only necessary to set aside 15-20 minutes each day. A simple meditation technique involves finding a quiet time and then to simply follow your breath flowing in and out. As soon as you notice your mind wandering, gently bring it back to the breath. It's that easy! It is also important to remember that making this quiet time a priority in your life is really about valuing yourself.

For many years I was very erratic with my meditation practices. Since committing to daily meditation time (which for me is early in the morning) I have found more emotional balance.

Things just don't seem to cause the reactive responses in

me that they once did. I guess you could call it a growing sense of inner peace. My morning meditation time is now a regular part of my life.

Chapter 8

Loving Your Body

A very special Hawaiian elder named Angeline Locey, the founder of a wonderful healing center on the island of Kauai, taught me about the importance of loving the body. She would always chant, "Malama Pono Ea Oi," as she lovingly massaged people's bodies. Translated it means, " I take back my body, I love my body." Over and over again, Angeline would remind everyone to love their bodies. She said that without the love for our bodies we can never be truly whole and healed.

Loving our body is certainly a challenge for most women. Our body seems to be our enemy. It's never quite perfect enough to please us. Somehow, the more we starve it, deny it and despise it, the more we add to our own self-hatred. How can it be otherwise? After all, we are our bodies. Learning to love and appreciate the uniqueness of our bodies, whatever the shape, characteristics or condition it may be in, is reclaiming the love for ourselves. And the secret is that the more we learn to love our bodies, the more they transform into the bodies we love!

There are many ways to begin loving your body. It can be as simple as indulging in a sensuous bath, complete with candles, music and aromatherapy bath oil. It is certainly a wonderful opportunity to relax and dissolve muscle tensions.

An aromatherapy body rub is another loving gesture. It is best done after a shower or bath. Add a few drops of your favorite aromatherapy oil into a capful of massage oil. Then with your finger tips gently massage the oil all over your body, beginning with the soles of the feet and moving all the way up to your head. Since you are using just a small amount of oil, it is quickly absorbed. As you massage, send loving thoughts to your body.

Other gestures of love may include receiving regular massages, taking time out in nature, afternoon naps, getting cuddles and eating nutritious foods. Discover your favorite ways or explore new ones. One thing is for sure, without learning to love your body, true inner harmony will always elude you.

Chapter 9

Emotional Healing and Spiritual Growth

Healing emotional pain is one of the purposes of this life time. It is called growth. We are truly blessed to be living in a time when we no longer need to keep our inner pain hidden away—eating away at our self-love, joy and creativity. Personal growth is becoming more widely accepted as a legitimate need of all people. There are so many wonderful resources presently available to anyone who truly desires to free themselves of the hurt of the past in order to live a more fulfilling life. Through the myriad of counselling techniques, seminars, classes, support groups, body work modalities, alternative healing methods and personal awareness books, tapes and videos, we are given countless opportunities to explore ourselves and shed old, outmoded ways of perceiving reality.

As women raised in a culture that has favored masculine values such as competition, hierarchy, control, rational thinking, obedience to authority and violence, we carry many wounds within us. These are the wounds handed down to us from the many past generations of women who were made to be silent, to feel powerless, guilt-ridden and worthless. Such emotional wounds blind us to the true beauty, wisdom and love of who we are. Perhaps the wide-spread disharmony presently manifesting within women's bodies is merely a reflection of generations who lived in denial of their Selves.

In Grace Gawler's book, *Women of Silence: The Emotional Healing of Breast Cancer*, she explores the hidden side of cancer—the emotional aspect of illness. "Although there are visible lumps on and in the body, these symptoms may actually have their origins within the soul where the creative threads of life dwell. When there are blocks in the creative flow of a woman's life and when the expression of that creativity is blocked, her creative knots can become knotted into what are unhealthy 'knots of the soul'. These 'knots' are formed by frustrated emotional energy at a very deep level of the psyche.

"Interestingly, women dealing with breast cancer almost always have a history of unresolved emotional pain throughout their life. These are the shackles that must be released."

As though awakening from a long sleep, women all over the world are returning to honor the wise woman within. Emotional healing is the path which leads to greater spiritual awareness—the awareness of a reality where all life is bound together with invisible threads of love.

Chapter 10

Coming Full Circle

Many thousands of years ago, forgotten by history but not by the memories in our bones, the feminine principle as embodied by women gave rise to the flourishing of the cultures where nature and all of life was recognized. Women were honored as representatives of nature's beauty, wisdom and the mysteries of life. It was a time when women were so finely attuned to life's secrets that they were the spiritual and political leaders, the healers, the artisans and educators.

As the full moon wanes, so too do all things. Not as decline and death but rather as change and growth. As the light of those feminine cultures was eclipsed by the new male-dominated world, all that was once held sacred became profane. The gifts and strengths of women were turned into weaknesses and faults. Women were defiled and perceived as less than human—and treated accordingly. Women learned to hate themselves and their bodies. Their only value came from either child bearing and child rearing or as sources of sexual pleasure.

But we now move once again slowly towards the light. We are coming to the end of this dark moon phase of history. It is no coincidence that women are rejecting all the ways that have usurped their true power and true instinctual wisdom.

Regaining an appreciation of her body is an essential part of a woman's re-awakening. While the Pill appeared at a time of history when women demanded their sexual freedom and independence, we now know, without a doubt, that the short-term benefits have demanded a terrible price. Filling our bodies with drugs that stopped our natural flow of hormones not only unbalanced our bodies, they also disconnected us from our feminine cyclic wisdom—the very heart and soul of a woman.

It is becoming evident that the Pill no longer serves the empowerment of women. It sounds a death knell—if not the death of women's bodies, surely the death of their spirit. It is only by embracing the wisdom of nature, natural cycles, natural medicines, natural foods and natural rhythms that women will once again find their wholeness and themselves. Successful and healthy contraception and conception are a part of woman's initiation into her own mystery which she has denied herself for so long.

Menopause is another initiation into women's mysteries. It does not need to be successfully 'managed'. It is not a disease condition that must be controlled or overcome. It does not, under normal conditions, necessitate drugs, surgery or manipulation of our bodies into unnatural processes. It is a rite of passage that all women must make. The need is for menopause to be a time for women to be honored, nurtured, understood and celebrated.

Real healing can only be attained by returning to inner balance, perhaps for the very first time in one's life. For so many years, the vast majority of women throughout the planet have lived their lives without realizing just how disconnected they were from themselves. There is much that we, as women, have forgotten about our innate wisdom and healing nature. There is also much that we have been taught to disdain about ourselves and our bodies. Now it is time to remember! It's time for the tying together of all the threads that weave the magnificent tapestry of a woman's wholeness. Life is beckoning us to return to balance for the sake of ourselves, our future generations and our planet.

PART FIVE

*How to Get Younger and Healthier
As We Get Older*

Updated 2009

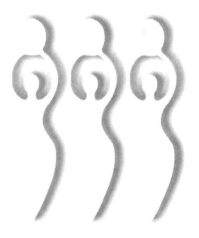

Chapter 1

Getting Younger and Healthier As We Get Older

When I first began to investigate the unfamiliar world of women's hormones, it was out of a desperate need to get my own hormones back on track. Just like in the classic movie, *The Wizard of Oz* when Toto pulls back the curtain revealing the real person controlling the levers of the Great Oz, I, too, had my "Oz Moment". With each area of women's health issues that I would research and investigate, I discovered deceit and the foisting of unproven or potentially harmful pharmaceutical or surgical solutions upon trusting women.

Why would such a thing happen? Well, it's no secret that women and women's health problems add substantial revenue to the coffers of Big Pharma.

I have always believed that women must have access to truthful information so they can make the most informed decisions possible.

So, I continued to write and share the discoveries that were being revealed to me. I have shed light on the myths and truths on many topics near and dear to women... osteoporosis, the Pill, hysterectomies, the new Cervical Cancer Vaccine, Gardasil, the endocrine disrupting hormones in the environment and in our tap water, the impact of cell phones on our hormones, the hidden agenda of Breast Cancer Awareness month...to name just a few.

When it came to my own health, to be quite honest, I initially didn't understand all the messages of distress my body was giving me. Although my personal encounter with anxiety attacks and particularly night sweats made me profoundly aware of the hormonal imbalances that were occurring in my body during my perimenopausal years. There were many other symptoms that eluded my understanding of what was happening. Like so many women, I learned to put up with the achy joints, depression, insomnia, chronic hayfever, eczema, a hypothyroid condition and increasing weight gain. It didn't even dawn on me at that time that I had chronic underlying health issues eroding my health.

It is easy to mistakenly interpret these symptoms as the burdensome price your pay for entering middles age!

Don't ever do that!

As I became more deeply involved with alternative and complementary medicine, I began to unravel the patterns behind these health issues which have really plagued me for most of my life.

As a health writer for many holistic health publications nationally and internationally, and as Senior editor of the well respected *Total Health Magazine*, I had many opportunities to research and write about subjects and proven holistic solutions for my health challenges.

The more I learned, the more I made the necessary changes through implementing dietary and life style changes, a nutritional protocol of vitamins, mineral and herbs and homeopathic remedies, the more my body healed. I also gathered a team of alternative medical doctors, acupuncturists and chiropractors to guide me in my rejuvenation process.

So, here I am many years down the track. I no longer suffer from hay fever, allergies, aches and pains, eczema, hypothyroidism, nor weight issues. I can honestly say that at this point in my life, my health is so much better than what it was when I first embarked on this path more than a decade ago.

Getting younger and healthier as I journey through my life is becoming a reality!

This is the future we can all create for ourselves.

In this new section of this revised and updated version of *Hormone Heresy*, I have included the additional information

that has been an important part of my own on-going self discovery and healing. The more health questions I had, the more
I researched and the more I learned.

These new chapters will further enlighten you to the many
important issues directly impacting your hormones and your
health. They also provide the opportunity to gaining more
knowledge about proven and safe health solutions.

I personally use the various products which I write about
in the following chapters. They have helped to change my life.
I invite you to keep an open mind and to discover what might
also be beneficial for your healing and rejuvenation.

But, no one walks the exact same path.

I have included a chapter with specific protocols for many
of women's health problems that I hope will assist you as a
guide on your healing path. There is also an extensive resource
section that can direct you to the products that may be a part
of the solution to your health challenge.

Our health is the most precious thing we have. The more
we seek knowledge, the more we will open ourselves to the
healing power found within nature and within ourselves. The
more we learn about our bodies and the influences that support
our health, the more we can make the responsible choices that
lead us to optimal wellbeing. And the more we trust our innate
Wisdom, the more we realize that we can, indeed, regenerate
and rejuvenate ourselves at any age.

In this new and more comprehensive edition of *Hormone
Heresy* are many of the keys that can lead you down the yellow
brick road of Life where you can, literally, become younger
and healthier as you get older.

Chapter 2

The Physiology of Hormones

Women and hormones equal big business these days. Like animals lured into a snare by a trail of crumbs, women have been cajoled with scientific studies, media advertising, patient hand books and drug samples to accept Hormone Replacement Therapy as a magic potion. HRT is praised as the cure for hot flashes and all the other symptoms assigned to the menopause pantheon. In addition, it is considered an anti-aging medicine acting as a talisman to ward off osteoporosis, heart disease and Alzheimer's.

Millions of menopausal women flock to their doctors' offices each year seeking relief from such complaints as hot flashes, night sweats, bloating, indigestion, allergies, head-aches, insomnia, fatigue, depression, high blood pressure, weight gain, head hair loss, facial hair growth, mood swings, aging skin, irritability, foggy thinking, lack of concentration, anxiety attacks, heart palpitations, bone loss and heavy bleed-ing. The common panacea prescribed for all these symptoms is usually HRT or a more recent trend, Bio-identical Hormone Replacement Therapy (BHRT). All these presenting symptoms are lumped together into the menopausal pigeonhole; estrogen deficiency is the diagnosis, and hormone replacement becomes the cure. It's an obvious and simple solution for hormonal imbalance—or so we are led to believe.

But what if these symptoms that mostly plague 40 and 50-year-old women are not at all about menopause? What if it's not estrogen deficiency but rather an imbalance between estrogen excess and progesterone deficiency that is the cause of these discomforts? What if the real physiological problems are, in fact, being ignored, misdiagnosed or misunderstood? And what if the pathological condition of "menopause," the supposed cause of a midlife woman's lament, doesn't even exist?

Unfortunately, women have been intentionally led on a merry hormone wild goose chase. While the pathologic medicating of menopausal women with potent, carcinogenic and dangerous steroid drugs has filled the coffers of the drug companies and doctors alike, the real cause of these health problems has been ignored... and so have safe and effective solutions. Menopause, far from being a stage in a woman's life that leads her into a dark dungeon of discomfort and decline, is actually a time when the abuses of lifestyle, poor diet, environmental toxicity, and stress finally take their toll.

Hormonal imbalances are, in fact, symptoms of poor health. If the symptoms are addressed only with various HRT formulations, the real underlying issues are not just ignored but in all likelihood, worsened.

Digestion, Malabsorption and Candida

A healthy digestive and gastrointestinal system are the keys to good health. It begins with the first bite. Proper digestion depends on the proper secretion of digestive enzymes and the digestive system's ability to assimilate and absorb foods. Most health problems begin here. No matter what foods are eaten, everything in our diet is composed of proteins, carbohydrates, fat, sugars and fiber. The essential digestive enzymes (protease, amylase, lipase, disaccharidase and cellulase) are necessary to break them down during digestion. Without adequate enzymes, people become intolerant to certain foods which leads to a whole host of food allergies. Without adequate enzymes, digestion is seriously impaired.

Enzyme deficiencies can exacerbate many health issues: a

compromised immune system, chronic infections, fluid retention, chronic constipation, hypoglycemia, moodiness, depression, irritability, anxiety, impaired bone metabolism leading to osteoporosis, blood clots, allergic reactions, diabetes, high cholesterol, high blood pressure and varicose veins.

Our modern lifestyle has contributed to the depletion of digestive enzymes. Enzymes are impaired by pesticides and chemicals, genetic engineering, food irradiation, hydrogenated oils, microwaves, radiation, fluoridation, heavy metals and mercury amalgams. Supplementing one's diet with plant-based digestive enzymes is becoming necessary for people of all ages. What make things worse is that after turning 40, the body naturally tends to produce less enzymes.

Another serious digestive problem is a condition called candidiasis or better known as candida. Approximately 1 in 3 American women suffer from this toxic yeast overgrowth caused by eating large amounts of sugar, prolonged or repeated use of antibiotics, birth control pills, estrogen therapy and cortisone. Candida has been found to produce 79 different toxins that are known to wreak havoc with the immune system.

There is a long list of symptoms associated with a candida overgrowth. They include depression, anxiety attacks, mood swings, lack of concentration, drowsiness, poor memory, headaches, insomnia, fatigue, bloating, constipation, bladder infections, menstrual cramps, vaginal itching, muscle and joint swelling, pain, hypothyroidism and skin problems.

To rid the body of pathological yeast and improve the immune system, it is important to:

❖ eliminate sugar in all its forms

❖ eliminate foods gluten foods

❖ eat organic foods

❖ use natural anti-fungal remedies such as grapefruit seed extract, oregano oil, probiotics (friendly bacteria), cultured foods and digestive enzymes.

It is obvious from the long list of above symptoms that so-called menopause affliction could be due to chronic digestive problems. And it is interesting to note that both the Pill and HRT cause impaired digestion and candida overgrowth. In fact, candida feeds on estrogens. And so the vicious cycle continues.

A Rise in Hypothyroidism

The thyroid gland is an important component of the immune system. It is a small butterfly-shaped endocrine organ at the base of the neck. The thyroid is the body's thermostat controlling body temperature, energy use, the rate which organs function and the speed with which the body uses food. The thyroid is implicated in the functioning of all body processes and organs.

Thyroid problems are also of epidemic proportion in women, 15-20 times more prevalent than in men. It is estimated that between 50-80 percent of Western women suffer from hypothyroidism, an underactive thyroid.

Hypothyroidism has a direct effect on women's hormonal health. Seventy percent of women with infertility and miscarriages have hypothyroidism. In addition, fibrocystic breast disease, fibroids, ovarian cysts, endometriosis, PMS, menopausal symptoms and multiple sclerosis are caused or worsened by an underactive thyroid. Other symptoms include fatigue, depression, weight gain, cold hands and feet, skin problems (itching, eczema, acne, dry and scaly), loss of memory, lack of concentration, migraines, muscle aches, swelling of eyelids, constipation, brittle nails and poor vision.

A deficiency of the thyroid hormone can also lead to elevated cholesterol and triglyceride levels, putting older women at greater risk of heart disease. Hypothyroidism weakens the immune system and makes women more susceptible to recurring infections.

While hypothyroidism is also one of the least understood health conditions by the medical profession, the causes are readily known by alternative medicine. Radiation is probably the greatest environmental cause. This includes both ionizing radiation emitted by nuclear reactors and non-ionizing radiation from the electromagnetic fields of common electrical appliances, cell phones and other wireless technologies and geopathic stress zones.

Another significant cause is estrogen dominance (an excess of estrogen in relation to progesterone). Estrogen dominance, which interferes with the uptake of thyroid hormones can result from taking birth control pills, estrogen replacement therapy, as well as exposure to pesticides, and other environmental toxins. Stress and nutritional deficiencies in selenium, glutathione, iodine and zinc also have a key role. And once again an imbalance in microflora of the gut decreases the body's ability to uptake thyroid hormone.

Other thyroid inhibitors include excess intake of unsaturated fats (liquid oils at room temperature), fluoride, heavy metal poisoning, mercury exposure (from amalgam fillings, vaccinations, fish and coal-burning plants), low protein diet, gluten and soy products, raw cruciferous vegetables (cabbage, cauliflower, broccoli, etc.) and dieting. The most popular thyroid medication, Synthroid, is an inactive form of the thyroid hormone that actually shrinks the thyroid gland, suppresses the pituitary and suppresses cellular respiration. Synthroid can also increase the risk of osteoporosis. The natural thyroid hormones such as Armour, Naturthroid or Westhroid provide the necessary T4 and T3 hormones.

We live in a thyroid-toxic culture and environment. No wonder hypothyroidism is such a common disorder. Yet here are very effective natural approaches that help in regulating the thyroid. Natural progesterone balances the thyroid-inhibiting effect of estrogen dominance as does supplementation with thyroid glandular extracts, enzyme therapy, and herbal formulas.

Dietary recommendations to support thyroid function include getting adequate protein, i.e. organic beef, poultry, eggs, fish, and cultured milk products such as kefir and yogurt.

Thyroid healing foods include those high in the B vitamins such as wheat germ, whole grains, nuts, seeds, dark greens, legumes and Brewer's yeast. Other foods that assist thyroid function include seaweed and wheat germ oil. The minerals selenium, iodine and magnesium are all essential for a healthy functioning thyroid.

Another great thyroid promoting food is organic coconut oil. There are two groups of saturated fats— medium and long-chain. Medium-chain saturates, found in non-hydrogenated coconut oil, do not clog arteries nor do they cause heart disease. Instead, medium-chain saturated fats convert into energy, do not store as fat and enable the body to metabolize fat efficiently. In addition, coconut oil acts as an anti-histamine, an anti-diabetic, an anti-infective and even an anticancer agent!

Unfortunately most of the standard thyroid tests often fail to pinpoint an underactive thyroid, leading physicians to make erroneous diagnoses. Subclinical conditions abound. However, there are effective self-diagnostic tests. Take an underarm temperature reading with a thermometer first thing in the morning for five consecutive days. It is even more effective when you keep your eyes open and have exposure to bright lights for half an hour before taking the test. But remember to stay in bed and remain inactive. A low-functioning thyroid will show an average temperature of under 97.5 F. Also check the resting pulse. Less than 85 beats per minute plus a low basal temperature may indicate hypothyroidism.

Another simple test is to paint an area approximately 2 inches in diameter on your thigh or belly with a 2 percent tincture of iodine. If the yellowish stain disappears in less than 24 hours, it indicates your body has an iodine deficiency. Seaweed, Celtic sea salt or an iodine supplement can help replenish iodine levels.

The Adrenal Glands

The glands which work hand in glove with the thyroid are the adrenal glands, two small prune-shaped glands that sit on top of the kidneys. Although small in size, they are very big in function. They are involved in:

- ❖ manufacturing 28 different hormones
- ❖ the digestion of food, especially carbohydrates and sugar
- ❖ the regulation of the body's minerals
- ❖ producing and maintaining the body's energy levels in conjunction with the thyroid
- ❖ producing hormones that monitor stress

Progesterone is a necessary raw material for producing adrenal gland hormones.

Prolonged stress, whether as a result of emotional, environmental or physical causes, is disastrous for the adrenals. Initially, it increases the output of the long-term stress hormone cortisol. Cortisol helps to regulate blood sugar, the movement of carbohydrates, proteins and fats in and out of the cells, inflammation and muscle function. Chronic stress causes chronically elevated levels of cortisol resulting in weight gain (especially around the midsection), blood sugar imbalances, thinning skin, muscle wasting, memory loss, high blood pressure, dizziness, hot flashes, excessive facial hair, and other masculinizing tendencies.

Overworked adrenals will eventually crash, leading to adrenal exhaustion, a condition in which the body is unable to maintain adequate production of adrenal hormones. Symptoms of overtaxed adrenals include:

- ❖ extreme fatigue such as in Chronic Fatigue Syndrome
- ❖ irritability
- ❖ inability to concentrate
- ❖ frustration

- insomnia
- anxiety
- addiction to either sweet or salty foods
- allergies
- nervousness
- depression
- PMS
- sensitivity to cold
- diabetes
- headache
- chronic low blood pressure.

Adrenal exhaustion creates havoc with the endocrine system. Many hormonal imbalances in women of all ages are caused by over-worked adrenal glands. Nutrients that have special importance to the adrenal glands are the B vitamins (especially B-5), vitamin C, proteins, magnesium, manganese, zinc, potassium, plant enzymes, adrenal extracts and the amino acids tyrosine and phenylalanine. Rest is the best when it comes to rebuilding the adrenals. And so is stress reduction. Shedding one's life of those stressful events, people, demands, high-pressure jobs as well as addressing unresolved emotional wounds is vital for healing the adrenal glands.

As more and more women awaken from the spell that has been cast upon them, it becomes apparent that menopause is not the enemy of their quality of life. Popping a hormone pill is certainly not the solution. Regaining the knowledge of their female physiology, reducing their hectic lives, honoring the needs of their bodies and returning to the healing power of natural foods and natural medicines is indeed the greatest challenge for women in this new millennium.

Chapter 3

How to Balance Your Menopausal Moods

On my journey through the uncharted seas of perimenopause I encountered some rather rough sailing. My days were filled with the swells and troughs of depression, tears, mood swings, irrational angry outbursts, lethargy and fatigue. My nights found me in turmoil with gripping anxiety and panic attacks along with soaking night sweats. Add to this, the unexplained weight gain and low libido and I knew something was seriously awry. My moods and my body seemed totally out of control. What was happening to me?

The emotional roller-coaster that accompanies premenstrual syndrome, perimenopause and menopause is most profoundly connected to the flow of two powerful hormones, estrogen and progesterone. Nature has designed estrogen and progesterone to be partners in a delicate balancing act. When that balance teeters in either one direction or another, a whole host of health problems ensues. When estrogen is out of balance with progesterone a condition called "estrogen dominance" occurs. The imbalance that results causes depression, mood swings, anxiety, irritability, anger, insomnia, fatigue, weight gain, bloating, mental fogginess, low libido and sore breasts.

Estrogen excess plays a huge role in creating PMS symptoms. Progesterone is the dominant hormone during the two weeks after ovulation. It's produced in amounts 200 times greater than estrogen at that time. However, due to the many stresses, nutritional deficiencies and eating indiscretions, estrogen levels can far exceed progesterone levels. The woes of PMS (including the wild emotional ride) are the result of this topsy-turvy hormone production.

Hormonal Imbalance

Far from deficiency in estrogen, the modern menopausal woman is also more likely to experience high levels of estrogen and low levels of progesterone, creating that all-too-familiar estrogen dominant profile. In fact, the World Health Organization (WHO) has reported that an overweight postmenopausal woman has more estrogen circulating through her body than a skinny premenopausal woman. Through the use of saliva testing, the most valid way to test hormone levels according to the WHO, the prevalence of estrogen dominance has been confirmed. Instead of estrogen deficiency, most women are really suffering from a progesterone deficiency.

Even perimenopause, a five to ten year journey of hormonal adjustments preceding menopause, is now recognized as a time when the body is making really high levels of estrogen along with low progesterone output due to irregular ovulations. According to Dr. Jerilynn Prior, professor of endocrinology at the University of British Columbia, the various symptoms of perimenopause are due to an excess of estrogen not a deficiency. Dr Prior's research has also discovered that more than 25 percent of young women in their 20s are not ovulating every month, although they continue to menstruate, leading to a month-long estrogen dominant condition which worsens PMS mood swings and other symptoms.

Avoid Steroids

When steroid hormones are used, either in the form of the pill or hormone replacement therapy (HRT) for PMS, perimenopause or menopause, estrogen levels may be raised by as much as 100 times more than what the body would normally be making. For many women, these treatments will not only create but will also worsen depression, anger flare-ups, anxiety, panic attacks, insomnia, lethargy and unpredictable mood swings. The pill and HRT also rob the body of vital nutrients such as vitamin B-complex, E, C, folic acid and zinc, which further compromises physical and emotional health.

In addition, estrogen blocks the release of hormones from the thyroid gland, contributing to a sluggish thyroid condition known as hypothyroidism. Symptoms of hypothyroidism include depression, postpartum depression, mood swings, lethargy, mental fogginess, weight gain and menstrual irregularities. Estrogen can also activate the adrenals to produce the stress hormone, cortisol, leading to various harmful effects, including brain aging and bone loss. Excessive demand placed on the adrenals will lead to adrenal exhaustion causing anxiety, panic attacks, depression or rapid mood swings, mental sluggishness, feeling mentally and physically over-stressed, crying bouts, insomnia, night sweats and generalized fatigue.

A woman's ability to feel and express her deep emotional life is one of the greatest gifts of being a woman. However, hormone balance is a delicate matter. Working long hours, getting too little sleep, daily stresses, a diet of too much sugar, caffeine, refined carbohydrates, alcohol and hydrogenated oils and skipping meals will all lead to estrogen dominance and its domino effect on the entire endocrine system.

Correct Underlying Problem

Whatever emotional imbalance a woman may be experiencing, it's a powerful signal to address the underlying imbalance. Although mood swings of whatever variety have many causes, hormonal balance is always a key component. It's important to work with a competent holistic practitioner to discover and correct the underlying health problem behind the emotional imbalance.

Popular drug therapies such as Prozac, Paxil, Zoloft and minor tranquilizers may only alleviate the symptoms, never the cause. They also have serious side effects which include mood swings, depression, anxiety, insomnia, hypertension weight gain, suicidal behavior and sexual dysfunction.

My perilous perimenopausal journey was a time of profound learning about my body and its hormonal transitions. With the assistance of my natural healing team of a traditional Chinese herbalist, chiropractor and holistic physician, I was able to navigate myself back to balance. I increased progesterone levels by using a transdermal natural progesterone cream. I gave my liver extra support by adding the herb milk thistle, the antioxidants vitamins A, C and E, coenzyme Q10 and alpha lipoic acid. Adding healthy portions of liver-friendly foods such as broccoli, Brussels sprouts, carrots, sweet potatoes, tomatoes, spinach and kale while reducing sugar, refined carbohydrates, gluten foods, caffeine, alcohol, preservatives and trans-fatty acids.

I also committed to a nutritional and herbal program and added more hormone-balancing foods such as whole grains, plenty of fresh organic vegetables and fruits, quality proteins, essential fatty acids and pure water. Regular exercise, meditation and personal quality time were given prominence in my stress reduction program. Within just a couple of months, my panic attacks permanently ceased, my mood swings disappeared, the night sweats ended, my energy increased, my sleeping was sound, my weight went down and libido went up. I realized that a woman's life doesn't need to be a journey of perpetual emotional storms.

Chapter 4

Natural Solutions for Healing Uterine Fibroids

I knew from the tension in Rosie's voice that something was wrong. She phoned me in a panic after her doctor told her that her heavy menstrual bleeding was caused by uterine fibroids. She was hoping to avoid the only option offered to her by her doctor—a hysterectomy.

Fibroids were a complete mystery to Rosie, as they are to many women. I reassured her that there were many ways to reduce, if not totally eliminate, fibroids. Before considering a hysterectomy, I encouraged her to incorporate a plan that included dietary and lifestyle changes as well as nutritional supplementation. She decided to give a more holistic approach a try.

Fibroids and Hormonal Imbalance

Fibroids are quite common and found in 20-30 percent of all women by the age of 40 and more than 40 percent of women have them by the time they reach menopause.

The most important fact about fibroids is that they are benign (non-cancerous) tumors. A fibroid is formed from excess fibrin (scar tissue), smooth muscle tissue, and generally, pockets of estrogen. They are found on and within the uterine wall or in the uterine cavity and can vary in size from being very small to weighing several pounds.

It is estimated that 75 percent of women are unaware that they have fibroids since they are symptom-free. The most common symptom of fibroids is heavy menstrual bleeding, often with large clots. Regular cycles of heavy bleeding can lead to anemia. The size or position of a fibroid can exert pressure on the bladder, bowels or sensitive pelvic nerves, causing a variety of symptoms including pelvic pain, frequent urination, constipation, low back pain, and irritable bowel.

Although fibroids are the number one reason that doctors perform a hysterectomy, there are, in fact, many effective, natural treatments that can successfully resolve fibroids.

Balance Hormones, Banish Fibroids

Fibroids are hormone dependent, thriving on estrogen. The primary cause of fibroids is a hormonal imbalance caused by an excess of estrogen and a deficiency of progesterone.

This estrogen "dominance" can be fuelled by many things including the use of "the Pill," fertility drugs, or hormone replacement therapy. Other contributing factors to estrogen excess include bowel toxicity, liver congestion, inflammation, heavy metal toxicity, hypothyroidism and exposure to environmental estrogens (e.g., organochlorine pesticides, pharmacologic compounds). From my clinical practice, I have also observed that stress from unresolved emotional conflicts regarding creativity, reproduction, and relationships can often exacerbate hormonal imbalances.

Since there is a direct relationship between fibroids and estrogen excess, restoring balance by increasing progesterone levels is necessary. Transdermal natural progesterone cream, a bio-identical source of progesterone, helps to restore this crucial balance. The recommended dose is 1/8 to 1/2 teaspoon rubbed twice daily (am and pm) on soft tissue such as the abdomen, inner arms, or inner thighs usually from day 13-26 of the menstrual cycle.

A standardized extract of the herb chaste tree berry (140 to 275 milligrams daily) has been shown to also increase progesterone levels. However, it may take three or four months before its full benefit is experienced.

In general, all foods that promote estrogen excess must be reduced or avoided: all non-organic, processed foods, dairy products, sugar, refined carbohydrates, unfermented soy products, alcohol, and coffee. Environmental estrogens are also found in personal care products, cosmetics, household cleaning products, plastics, and all forms of pesticides. Whenever possible, use only organic chemical-free products.

Fibroids and Your Liver

The liver plays an important role in hormonal balance. Estrogen is deactivated by the liver before being eliminated from the body. Liver problems and liver congestion will raise levels of circulating estrogen and thus aggravate fibroid growth. A vitamin B-complex (100 mg) helps support the liver by enabling it to break down estrogens while vitamin E (600 IU) will regulate bleeding and normalize estrogen levels.

Indole-3-carbinole (150 to 300 mg daily), an active ingredient of cruciferous vegetables such as broccoli, Brussels sprouts, cabbage and cauliflower, has a powerful effect on the liver's ability to properly metabolize estrogens. The supplement Calcium D-glucarate (150 to 300 mg daily), a natural substance found in many fruits and vegetables clears estrogens and xeno-estrogens out of the body. Liver support herbs such as milk thistle, dandelion, goldenseal, barberry, and artichoke detoxify a wide range of hormones, drugs, and toxins. The B-compound vitamins, choline, inositol, and methionine, are excellent for liver cleansing.

Regular exercise is essential to help reduce the growth of fibroids.

Once released from the liver into the small and large intestines, estrogen may be reabsorbed back into the body if the intestines are sluggish. Since slow transit time and constipation increases estrogen levels—increasing water consumption, fiber intake, and taking bowel-cleansing herbs will aid proper elimination.

The Benefits of Castor Oil Packs and Coffee Enemas

Two other effective strategies for eliminating fibroids includes the use of castor oil packs to increase healthy circulation of the pelvic cavity and weekly use of coffee enemas for liver detoxification.

Castor oil has a long history of traditional medical use dating back to ancient Egypt. Castor oil is derived from the castor bean (*Ricinus communis*).

Castor oil appears to have a unique ability to sink transdermally (through the skin) to relax smooth muscle. This simple mechanical action has a beneficial influence on all hollow organs, specifically the blood and lymph vessels, the uterus, fallopian tubes, bowels, gall bladder, and even the liver (which is not hollow but is filled with venous lakes).

A castor oil pack is placed on the skin to increase circulation and to promote elimination and healing of the tissues and organs underneath the skin. It is often used to stimulate the liver, relieve pain, increase lymphatic circulation, reduce inflammation and improve digestion.

Castor oil packs have many applications, and are specific in cases of uterine fibroids and ovarian cysts that are not cancerous. Packs also relieve ovarian pain or help with healing after a ruptured ovarian cyst. Other conditions that respond to castor oil packs include headaches, liver disorders, constipation, intestinal disorders, gallbladder inflammation or stones, and conditions with poor elimination.

Castor oil packs are made by soaking a piece of flannel in castor oil and placing it on the abdomen. The flannel is covered with a sheet of plastic, and then a hot water bottle or heating pad is placed over the plastic to heat the pack.

Castor oil application increases the efficiency of circulation through your pelvis in general. Good circulation is required for supportive nutrients to be delivered to the cells, and for waste products and inflammatory factors to be removed. If a castor oil pack is placed over your liver area, it will help your liver to do its work more efficiently, including the metabolism of your hormones.

To be effective, a castor oil pack must be used at least 3 times a week for at least 30-60 minutes, although 5 times a week is better. In cases of long-term chronic pain, it works best to commit to a 6 week treatment period using a castor oil pack 5 times per week, then as needed for episodes of pain.

Always choose a high quality castor oil and use cotton or wool flannel cloths if possible.

The purpose of a coffee enema is to help detoxify the liver! Enemas and colonics have been used for hundreds of years. Coffee enemas have a chemical makeup that is stimulative. The enzymes in coffee, known as palmitates, help the liver carry away the toxins in bile acid. The coffee is absorbed into the hemorrhoidal vein, then taken up to the liver by the portal vein. With the bile ducts dilated, bile carries toxins away to the gastrointestinal tract. Simultaneously, peristaltic activity is encouraged because of the flooding of the lower colon. Thus, when the colon is evacuated, the toxins and bile are carried out of the body.

The coffee enema is safe even for people who are sensitive to caffeine because the coffee remains in the sigmoid colon, where it will not be absorbed, provided the proper amount is used and the enema bag is not placed too high.

Using a coffee enema twice a week to help reduce the size of a fibroid is recommended. However it can be used more frequently. After the fibroid has shrunk, a coffee enema is a great liver detox to do once or twice a month.

Coffee Enema Recipe

Bring 8 cups of water to a boil.

Grind eight heaping spoonfuls of organic coffee. Put it in a french press pot. You can use a drip coffee maker, but be sure to use organic, non-bleached coffee filters.

Pour the water over the coffee grounds and let it steep then cool for one hour or more.

After this amount of time, the liquid should be about body temperature. If you stick your finger in the water it should be lukewarm or cool, but not hot.

Press the coffee grounds to the bottom, then pour the coffee liquid into the enema bag.

Never utilize flavored coffee, sweetened coffee, or coffee with milk (cafe au lait) for this purpose.

The Thyroid – Fibroid Connection

There is also a relationship between a sluggish thyroid and fibroids. So, it is important to assess thyroid function. A blood test is usually recommended. In addition, I suggest taking your first morning temperature, before getting out of bed. A consistent reading of 97.6 F or below indicates a low functioning thyroid.

In hypothyroidism, there is increased activity of the pituitary gland aimed at trying to stimulate the thyroid to produce more hormone secretions, and the increased pituitary activity may spill over to affect the ovaries and increase their estrogen output. Unless the health of the thyroid is considered in assessing any "female" complaint, a major contributing factor may be overlooked.

Other Useful Strategies

Since fibroids are composed of fibrin, or scar tissues, the protein-dissolving action of a systemic oral enzyme such a Serrapeptase (5 tablets 3x daily an hour before or 2 hours after meals) has the ability to actually dissolve the hard, fibrous material of a fibroid. Serrapeptase also exerts extremely high anti-inflammatory properties, a condition associated with fibroids.

The herb, Shepherd's purse is used to stop heavy bleeding and hemorrhaging, particularly from the uterus and is considered most effective for treating chronic uterine bleeding disorders from fibroids.

Successfully healing any health problem often requires the assistance of qualified holistic heath practitioners trained at finding the root causes of fibroids. The following modalities are effective in treating fibroids: acupuncture and Chinese herbs, naturopathy, homeopathy, Western herbal medicine, and chiropractic.

If at all possible, it is important to resolve fibroids when they're small. Larger fibroids are more difficult to successfully treat.

Determined to avoid a hysterectomy, Rosie committed herself wholeheartedly, to a healing program. By improving her diet, using nutritional support, detoxifying her body and reducing stress, she successful stopped the heavy bleeding, shrank her fibroids and kept her uterus!

Chapter 5

Hysterectomies – A Surgical Assault of Women

A woman's uterus and ovaries represent the essence of her feminine self. The uterus is the womb of life while the ovaries are the fundamental reproductive organs pumping out the three key sex hormones, progesterone, estrogen and testosterone. However, there is much more to these dynamic organs than has been previously thought.

These reproductive organs have another vital role. The uterus and ovaries are related to a woman's innermost sense of self and her inner world. It reflects her inner emotional reality and her belief in herself at the deepest level. They are the center of a woman's creative self.

Aside from the ovary's function of storing and maturing the eggs, it has another important role as an endocrine gland which produces hormones before, during and after menopause. Far from the popular myth that ovaries dry out, shrivel up and become completely useless at menopause, the ovaries continue to function throughout a woman's life.

Considering the immense significance of the uterus and ovaries to the life of a woman, it is a rather shocking fact that a hysterectomy is the number one surgical procedure for women.

How popular? In the U.S. more than 620,000 hysterectomies are performed each year. One out of three women will have had a surgical menopause, a hysterectomy that includes removal of the uterus and ovaries, before 60 years of age. To date about 22 million American women have had their uteri removed.

Are hysterectomies really necessary? According to Dr. Stanley West, chief of reproductive endocrinology at St. Vincent's Hospital, New York, "more than 90 percent of hysterectomies are unnecessary. Worse still, the surgery can have long-lasting physical, emotional and sexual consequences that may seriously undermine a woman's health and well-being."

Since the vast majority of hysterectomies are not truly medically imperative, it is stunning how often dietary and nutritional support and healing modalities such as acupuncture, lifestyle changes, detoxification, stress management techniques and emotional/spiritual approaches can heal the vast majority of these problems.

What is A Hysterectomy?

A hysterectomy is, by definition, the removal of a vital female organ, the uterus. However, more than 40 percent of the time perfectly healthy ovaries are also removed. The fallopian tubes and cervix are sometimes removed as well. The term "total hysterectomy" is now popularly used to describe the removal of the uterus, ovaries, fallopian tubes and part of the cervix.

More than 75 percent of hysterectomies are performed on women between the ages of 20 and 49. The older the woman is when undergoing a hysterectomy, the more likely that she will also have her perfectly healthy ovaries removed as a preventative measure.

The consequences of losing one's ovaries cannot be overstated. Premenopausal women will undergo an "instant" menopause, complete with symptoms that are far more severe than those that accompany normal menopause, which follows a natural adjustment in hormone production. The rationale for removing the ovaries during a hysterectomy is to prevent ovarian cancer which, in fact, only affects about one percent of women. And even then, the risk of ovarian cancer is not totally eliminated because ovarian tissue still remains. Without her ovaries a woman will forever be at a greater risk for both osteoporosis and heart disease, both of which represent a far greater statistical threat than ovarian cancer.

Why Have One?

A hysterectomy is offered as a treatment for several conditions. The leading cause is uterine fibroids, benign growths that, while sometimes troublesome and painful, are not life threatening. Fibroids account for about 30 percent of all hysterectomies. Endometriosis ranks second and leads to about 24 percent of all hysterectomies. The third-ranking indication is a prolapsed uterus caused by the loosening of the muscular supports. Prolapses account for about 20 percent. Endometrial hyperplasia (abnormal proliferation of cells in the endometrium due to excessive estrogen stimulation) ranks fourth at six percent. The remaining include menstrual disorders, ovarian cysts and pelvic inflammatory disease.

Only 10 percent of all hysterectomies are due to cancer. According to Dr. West, "Chances are that you are in the 90 percent, not the 10 percent." He believes that the only 100 percent appropriate reason for performing a hysterectomy is cancer of the reproductive organs.

While a hysterectomy is a fairly simple operation that involves detaching the uterus from the ligaments that support it and the blood vessels, it is far from safe. Up to one-half of all patients develop complications, some of which can be quite serious. Many of these complications are the preventable outcome of sloppy surgery and may involve adhesions, infections and damage to the bladder, bowel and uterus. Postoperative bleeding can lead to fatal hemorrhaging. An alarming statistic is that one out of 1000 patients will die.

The Side-effects

The after effects of a hysterectomy are most dramatic. In a relatively short period of time a woman may experience fatigue, insomnia, urinary problems, headaches, dizziness, vertigo, nervousness, irritability, anxiety, heart palpitations, joint pain, weight gain, vaginal dryness, diminished physical strength, difficult or painful sexual intercourse, hair loss and a variety of skin problems.

The incidence of post-hysterectomy depression appears relatively widespread. Dr. Susan Love, author of *Dr. Susan Love's Hormone Book*, states that some 30 to 50 percent of women suffer from depression while some other researchers estimate that this number may be as high as 70 percent. For some it is minor and short lived while for others it becomes a chronic state. Other psychological disturbances include mood change, anxiety and irritability. The hormonal disruptions brought on by the surgery can be far-reaching, affecting the nerve and hormone interactions responsible for a sense of emotional well-being.

Without the uterus holding the other pelvic cavity organs in place, there is a tendency for the bowel and bladder to prolapse. After a hysterectomy, the hip bones tend to widen, causing back, leg and foot problems.

What Women Aren't Being Told

The uterus is far from a disposable organ. It makes a little known hormone called prostacyclin which protects against heart disease and unwanted blood clotting. Since prostacyclin cannot be synthetically manufactured, once the uterus is removed its protective benefits are gone forever.

The uterus also is an important sex organ. The accelerating pitch of sexual excitement prompts the uterus to contract and rise out of the vagina. At orgasm, it undergoes a series of contractions. All the other so-called orgasms—vaginal, clitoral and nipple—are the initiators of sexual excitement but uterine contractions are the end point of this excitement. The female orgasm requires these contractions. Without a uterus, orgasm can be difficult to achieve.

A hysterectomy may also sever some of the nerves which go to the abdomen, the clitoris and the upper thigh. This can lead to a loss of tactile sensation from the waist to the mid-thigh region. Given these findings, there is no doubt that the loss of libido that is often reported after a hysterectomy is real, not imagined.

The medical terminology for removal of the ovaries (or testicles) is castration. No man in his right mind would ever consider having his testicles removed unless his life was seriously endangered. He certainly would never believe any doctor who told him this procedure would enhance his sex life. Yet gynecologists routinely encourage the removal of healthy ovaries and then promise women that their sex lives will be better than ever. It is therefore imperative for women to understand that their uteri and/or ovaries should not be willingly sacrificed until all other avenues have been thoroughly explored.

Women who have their uteri removed will automatically be put on some form of estrogen, usually a patch. This is, indeed, a most curious treatment since the uterus does not produce estrogen. In fact, the two leading reasons for a hysterectomy, fibroids and endometriosis, are conditions known to be caused or exacerbated by an excess of estrogen. Removing an organ that is an expression of an underlying imbalance will never resolve the problem. In this case, adding estrogen supplementation can create or even worsen health problems which include weight gain, depression, fluid retention, immune and autoimmune dysfunction, thyroid problems, migraines, foggy memory, breast cancer, liver and gall bladder disease and blood clots.

Estrogen should always be used with bio-identical progesterone to help restore hormonal balance.

Regaining Control Over Our Bodies

There is no doubt that there are valid and justified reasons for having a hysterectomy. Women who have been suffering from chronic, painful and sometimes life-threatening conditions have indeed benefited immensely from surgery. It is crucial, however, that every woman is adequately educated about the risks as well as the many alternative treatments. After all, common sense tells us that it is impossible to just pluck out an organ or disturb the body's balance without paying a price.

For those women who have already undergone hysterectomies, there is much that a woman can do to insure her health and well-being. For many women, estrogen is not even a necessary treatment. However, since a hysterectomy does increase the risk of a variety of health concerns, it is imperative that women seek guidance and treatment from qualified holistic health practitioners and be committed to making the appropriate lifestyle and dietary changes.

Perhaps the best advice for women facing the decision of a hysterectomy comes from Dr. West: "The challenge informed women face is to persuade doctors to turn away from the panaceas of the past to the treatments of the future. The last few decades have shown how forceful and resourceful women can be in pursuit of the economic and political power they were so long denied. Just as basic to full autonomy, is the control of your body and the right to make decisions about your health and health care on the basis of all available information, free from pressure, scare tactics and outdated doctor-knows-best paternalism. It is time we doctors stopped disassembling healthy women. But nothing will change until more women look their doctors in the eye and calmly state their determination to remain intact women."

FACTS ABOUT A HYSTERECTOMY

- ❖ Women may experience a loss of physical sexual sensation.

- ❖ A woman's vagina is shortened, scarred and dislocated by hysterectomy.

- ❖ Hysterectomy's damage is life-long. Among its most common consequences, in addition to operative injuries, are:

  - ❖ heart disease

  - ❖ osteoporosis

  - ❖ bone, joint and muscle pain and immobility

  - ❖ painful intercourse, vaginal damage

  - ❖ displacement of bladder, bowel and other pelvic organs

  - ❖ urinary tract infections, frequency of urination, incontinence

  - ❖ chronic constipation and digestive disorders

  - ❖ altered body odor

  - ❖ loss of short-term memory

  - ❖ blunting of emotions, personality changes, despondency, irritability, anger, reclusiveness and suicidal thinking.

- ❖ No drugs or other treatments can replace ovarian or uterine hormones or functions. The loss is permanent.

- ❖ Most women are castrated (removal of ovaries) at hysterectomy.

- ❖ Twice as many women in their 20s and 30s are hysterectomized as women in their 50s and 60s.

Chapter 6

Osteoporosis: The Bones of Contention

Osteoporosis is big news, and big business, these days. As a disease, it emerged out of obscurity only two decades ago to become a concern for women throughout the industrialized world. Advertising campaigns in the media and fact sheets in doctors' waiting rooms and pharmacies continually warn women of the dangers of disappearing bone mass.

The marketing hype announces that one woman in two over the age of 60 is likely to crumble from an osteoporotic fracture (yet one man in three will also get osteoporosis); that the incidence of hip fracture exceeds that of cancer of the breast, cervix and uterus combined; and that 16 percent of patients suffering hip fractures will die within six months while 50 percent will require long-term nursing care.

The statistics also say that in the United States more than 20 million people have osteoporosis and approximately 1.3 million people each year will suffer a bone fracture as a result of osteoporosis. In 1993, the US incurred an estimated loss of $10 billion due to lost productivity and health-care costs related to osteoporosis.

It's important to put these statistics into perspective. While it is true that death occurs in men and women who have hip fractures, these people are usually very elderly and frail. People who die from hip fractures are not only the most frail, but are also ailing from other causes.

Women are constantly bombarded with the message that

the war on bone loss must include calcium supplements and a daily consumption of calcium-rich foods, primarily dairy products. In spite of increased breast cancer risk, doctors continue to recommend long-term use of synthetic estrogen to the postmenopausal woman, and, if additional help is required, suggest use of bisphosphonate drugs like Fosamax, Boniva or Actonel. So, armed with this powerful arsenal, a woman is assured that she will walk tall and fracture-free through the latter part of her life. Unfortunately, this is far from the truth.

The most popular treatments for osteoporosis are in fact dangerous to women's health. Synthetic estrogen is a known carcinogenic drug. Most calcium supplements are not only ineffectual in rebuilding bone, but they can actually lead to mineral deficiencies, calcification in places like the arteries brain, breast or kidneys. And contrary to popular belief, dairy products have been proven to contribute to bone loss.

The Bare Bones About Bones

To understand the many myths about osteoporosis and its prescribed treatments, it is vital to understand the nature of bones. Bone is living tissue that undergoes constant transformation. Bone might appear to be static, but its basic components are continually renewed. At any given moment in each of us, there are from 1 to 10 million sites where small segments of old bone are being dissolved and new bone is being laid down to replace it. Bone tissue is nourished and detoxified by blood vessels in constant exchange with the whole body. A healthy body will ensure healthy bones.

Bone-forming cells are of two different kinds: osteoclasts and osteoblasts. The job of osteoclasts is to travel through the bone in search of old bone that is in need of renewal. Osteoclasts dissolve bone and leave behind tiny unfilled spaces. Osteoblast cells then move into these spaces in order to build new bone. This self-repair capability is extremely important. Imbalances in bone remodeling contribute to osteoporosis. When more old bone is eaten up than new bone is laid down, bone loss occurs.

Bone turnover never stops completely. In fact, after about the age of 50 the rate increases, though it's not quite co-coordinated. The bone-building cells, the osteoblasts, become less capable of refilling the spaces made by the osteoclasts. The peak amount of bone you started with and the rate of this loss determines the density of your bones. Density varies greatly in different individuals, cultures, races and sexes.

As Dr. Susan Love, author of *Dr. Susan Love's Hormone Book*, explains: "...the correct term for low bone density is 'osteopenia.' It is only one factor in osteoporosis and the fractures that result from it. Another factor is the micro-architecture of the bone. As osteoclasts absorb more bone than is rebuilt, the micro-architecture becomes fragile. As it weakens, the wrist and hip become more vulnerable to fracture. Your vertebra doesn't really fracture or crack but collapses on itself causing loss of height and, if enough vertebra are crushed, a dowager hump is created."

How real is this "dowager hump" syndrome? According to Dr. Bruce Ettinger, Associate Clinical Professor of Medicine at the University of California "...women shouldn't worry about osteoporosis. The osteoporosis that causes pain and disability is a very rare disease. Only 5 to 7 percent of 70-year-olds will show vertebral collapse; only half of these will have two involved vertebrae; and perhaps one-fifth or one-sixth will have symptoms. I have a very big referral practice and I have very few bent-over patients. There's been a tremendous hullabaloo lately, and there are a lot of worried women, and excessive testing and administration of medications."

The medical definition of osteoporosis used to be "fractures caused by thin bones." It has been redefined to "a disease characterized by low bone mass and micro-architectural deterioration of bone tissue which leads to increased bone fragility and a consequent increase in fracture risk." There is a problem with defining osteoporosis as a disease, not a fracture. Low bone mass is only one risk factor for osteoporosis, not osteoporosis itself. It's a warning sign that might be useful, so you can begin to consider ways to keep the disease itself from occurring.

Dr. Love offers a striking analogy: "This is like defining heart disease as having high cholesterol rather than having a heart attack. Needless to say, this new definition has increased the number of women and men who have osteoporosis."

Although this new disease has two components—bone mass and micro-architecture—micro-architecture is virtually ignored. The problem is that only bone density can be measured. And not everyone with low bone density will get fractures. For instance, Asian women have low bone density yet have very low rates of bone fractures.

The general assumption has been that once bone reaches a certain level of thinness, it becomes subject to fractures more easily. Now that more is known about bone physiology, it is clear that this is not the full story. Bone does not fracture due to thinness alone. Leading bone expert and author of *Better Bones, Better Body,* Susan E. Brown, PhD, states: "Osteoporosis by itself does not cause bone fractures. This is documented simply by the fact that half of the population with thin osteoporotic bones in fact never fracture."

Lawrence Melton of the Mayo Clinic noted as early as 1988: "Osteoporosis alone may not be sufficient to produce such osteoporotic fracture, since many individuals remain fracture-free even within the sub-groups of lowest bone density. Most women aged 65 and over and men 75 and over have lost enough bone to place them at significant risk of osteoporosis, yet many never fracture any bones at all. By age 80, virtually all women in the United States are osteoporotic with regard to their hip bone density, yet only a small percentage of them suffer hip fractures."

Why does there seem to be many more women now with osteoporosis than in the past? The level of bone density that defines osteoporosis has been set rather high, with the result that most older women will fall into the 'disease' category—which is very nice for the people in the business of treating disease.

The Bone-Building Drugs Scam – Beware of Fosamax

The drug companies boast one other weapon in their anti-osteoporosis arsenal: medication to halt bone loss. This is a class of drugs called bisphosphonates. They are more commonly known as Fosamax, Boniva and Actonel. Studies of this drug were cleverly stopped after four to six years. This is just the point at which the fracture rate for women taking similar drugs began to rise. So, although Fosamax will superficially appear to increase bone density, in reality it decreases bone strength. Bisphosphonates are a metabolic poison and will actually kill osteoclast cells that are required to maintain dynamic bone equilibrium.

In addition, they can cause severe and permanent damage to the jaw bone. Patients taking oral Fosamax began reporting deterioration of their jaw bones, known as osteonecrosis of the jaw.

Ever wonder why the instructions for taking any bisphosphonates warn against lying down for 30 minutes after taking it? That is because bisphosphonates can cause erosion of the cells of the esophagus and stomach leading to painful ulcerations.

These drugs are also hard on the kidneys and can cause diarrhea, flatulence, rashes, headaches and muscular pain. In addition, they cause deficiencies of calcium, magnesium and vitamin D, all essential for the bone-building process.

There are further problems with bisphosphonate drugs. They are a caustic chemical damaging any human tissue they come in contact with. They have been proven to induce inflammation by direct contact with body surfaces and they have been proven to set in motion a chain reaction of inflammatory events. It has been proven beyond any doubt that these drugs cause swollen bone due to their highly inflammatory nature. The FDA is now warning that at some point while taking these drugs there can be intense and even debilitating pain. This is obviously due to the caustic and highly inflammatory nature of these drugs.

Since October 2007 the FDA has also announced that it is reviewing the link between bisphosphonate drugs and atrial fibrillation. A new type of powerful bisphosphonate that involves a once a year intravenous infusion about to be released has shown a 150 percent increased risk for atrial fibrillation.

Atrial fibrillation is not the only potential cardiovascular risk. Science shows that bisphosphonates activate adhesion molecules, which are known to initiate plaque formation in arteries. A mouse study shows that bisphosphonates trigger the rupturing of atherosclerotic plaque—which causes strokes and heart attacks in humans.

Building Healthy Bones

It is clear that the osteoporosis treatments doctors most often recommend to women (HRT, calcium supplements, dairy products and drugs) have certainly benefited the medical establishment and drug companies most of all. The real long-term benefit to women is minimal at best, and life threatening at worst.

Fortunately there are other options that not only can prevent further deterioration of bone density and poor bone repair but also can actually increase bone mass in women of all ages. The six intervention areas that form the strongest, surest program for building and repairing bone include: maximizing nutrient intake, building digestive strength, minimizing anti-nutritive intake, exercising (especially with weights), developing an alkaline diet and promoting endocrine vitality. No matter where you are on the bone health continuum, no matter what your lifestyle has been, it is never too late to begin rebuilding healthy bones.

Some of the leading lights in safely preventing, halting and restoring bone mass include supplementation with natural progesterone, hydroxyapaptite, magnesium, boron, silicon, Vitamin D3 and Vitamin K-2. In fact, there are more than 20 key building nutrients that are required to ensure healthy bones.

Regular weight-bearing exercise program helps to increase

bone density. A woman's lifelong tendency to diet has been an unrecognized cause of bone loss. At least seven well-controlled studies have shown that when a woman diets and loses weight, she also loses bone. A recent study found that in less than 22 months, women who exercised three times a week increased their bone density by 5.2 percent, while sedentary women actually lost 1.2 percent. Effective strength training exercise includes such exercise as walking uphill, bicycling in low gear, climbing steps and training with weights.

Osteoporosis is not an aging disease or an estrogen or calcium deficiency but a degenerative disease of Western culture. We have brought it upon ourselves through poor dietary habits and lifestyle factors, and exposure to pharmaceutical drugs. It is our ignorance that has made us vulnerable to the vested interests that have intentionally distorted the facts and willingly sacrificed the health of millions of women at the altar of profit and greed. It is only by our willingness to take responsibility for our bodies and make the commitment to return to a healthy, balanced way of life that we'll be able to walk tall and strong for the rest of our lives.

Chapter 7

The Ancient Secret for Hormonal Balance

The immortal words of Hippocrates, the father of modern medicine, "Let your food be your medicine, and your medicine be your food" have never been a truer when it comes to hormonal health. The healing power of Nature has always provided the balm to restore health and balance, especially concerning hormones.

One of the gifts of Nature that has a very long tradition of being a powerful medicinal food is the Pomegranate. Mankind has revered the magical, mystical pomegranate since the dawn of recorded history. Ancient Greeks, Romans, and the peoples of China, India and the Middle East found its properties to be life-giving and invigorating.

Furthermore, the pomegranate fruit has been revered for thousands of years in all the world's major religions as The Fruit of Life, springing from The Garden of Paradise. As the traditional symbol of fertility and rebirth, it was also thought to bestow invincibility upon the person who enjoyed its glittering sweet tartness. It is a fruit of legend and power—a sacred symbol of human civilization.

This fruit, known as the "jewel of winter," was used for centuries in Middle Eastern folk medicine to treat many symptoms. Modern science has now shown that pomegranates contain a rich and diverse range of beneficial and protective substances, including phytoestrogens, polyphenols, ellagitannins, and anthocyanins. These compounds are powerful antioxidants. In fact, it is difficult to find a body part that is not supported by pomegranates. Recent studies demonstrate that pomegranates can:

* Support healthy cardiovascular system
  (heart, veins, blood and arteries)
* Support brain health
* Support liver health
* Support stomach health
* Support immune health
* Support healthy lipid levels in people with diabetes
* Support bone health
* Support oral health
* Support skin health
* Support prostate health

The Pomegranate, A Woman's Elixir

Traditionally the pomegranate has been renowned for being one of the most powerful elixirs for women's health, hormonal balance, beauty and fertility.

In herbal tradition there is a guiding principle called "The Doctrine of Signatures"— relating specifically to the similarity of plants (and their medicinal uses) to parts of the body. By careful observation one can intuit the healing properties of a plant from some aspect of its 'nature,' appearance, or place of growing. According to the renown Greek healer, Galen, this is "the ancient idea that the Creator left a signature on the plants to tell you what they're for."

Applying this, the Doctrine of Signatures can give greater appreciation about the correlation between the pomegranate's color and form and its corresponding medicinal properties. The reddish, round fruit is filled with its many arils (seeds surrounded by fluid filled sacs). These arils are encased within delicate inner membranes, very similar to the order, structure and appearance of the milk glands within the breast.

The pomegranate also reminds us of the shape and structure of the ovaries, with its many follicles. There is another correlation with the similarity of the color and shape of the heart and with the red juice reminiscent of the blood.

Far from just a quaint notion, modern science has actually discovered that the benefits of the pomegranate from its seeds, juice, peel, flowers and stem, do indeed have a profound impact on breast health, fertility, hormonal balance, skin rejuvenation and heart health.

The Pomegranate, Hormones and Menopause

What particularly intrigues scientists is the unique biochemistry of the pomegranate tree. The flowers, peel, juice and pericarp (the ripened walls of the plant's ovary) all contain compounds that especially help to support and modulate hormones and hormonal balance.

One of the most powerful parts of this plant is oil extracted from its tiny seeds. It takes 500 pounds of pomegranates to make just one pound of the oil. But the effort is definitely worth it. It turns out that pomegranate seed oil contains the greatest variety of phytoestrogens found anywhere in nature.

About 80 percent of the oil contains of a very rare fatty acid, known as punicic acid. Punic acid is similar to conjugated linoleic acid (CLA), which has potent fat burning abilities as well as anti-inflammatory effects. Not surprising, the conjugated fatty acids in pomegranate seed oil including, but not limited to punicic acid, also exhibit estrogenic properties.

In 1966, it was discovered that the seeds have the highest plant source of the estrogen, estrone. More recently, it was found that the main steroidal estrogen in pomegranate seed oil was 17 *alpha*-estradiol, a "bio-identical" estrogen that is hundreds of times weaker (and safer) than other forms of estrogen. In fact, 17 *alpha*-estradiol is the mildest of all steroidal estrogens.

The wide variety of safe phytoestrogens makes the pomegranate unique. Not only does it contain a wider range of phytoestrogens than any other plant, the estrogenic richness of pomegranate encompasses additional steroidal estrogens, such as estradiol, estriol and estrone with an assortment of many phytoestrogenic flavonoids.

There is even more goods news when it comes to pomegranates support of hormone health. The leaves of the pomegranate are one of the rare plant foods that contain apigenin, a progesterone-like compound with a calming, anti-anxiety and anti-depressive effect.

Dr. Ephraim Lanksy, one of world's leading researchers and experts in the health benefits of pomegranates has discovered that, "The entire fruit is laced with estrogens of various potencies in varying amounts. The mildest forms are the most common while the strongest kind is the rarest. There are over 10 estrogenic compounds found in the pomegranate fruit. Estrogen is defined as anything that binds to estrogen receptors. The forms that can bind but not stimulate a strong estrogenic effect are considered anti-estrogenic and prevent stronger from having an effect. This is important for modulating diseases that are provoked by too much estrogen."

The ability of the many components found in the pomegranate fruit to help safely modulate and regulate hormones is certainly good news for women of all ages. These weaker and safer forms of estrogens, (while helping to stimulate the less responsive menopausal estrogen receptors) will not contribute to estrogen dominance. Pomegranate's oil, as well as its juice, peel and flowers all help reduce many of the symptoms of hormonal imbalance. With the added progesterone-like benefits, women can experience more balanced hormones. The pomegranate assists women of all ages—it enhances fertility, balances menstrual cycles and corrects PMS. It also helps alleviate hot flashes, night sweats and other hormonal disturbances of perimenopausal and menopausal women.

Another challenge to women's health is the increasing incidence of chronic inflammation. Inflammatory conditions include: endometriosis, fibroids, polycystic ovarian syndrome, arthritis, autoimmune disease, asthma, metabolic syndrome, diabetes cardiovascular disease and even cancer. Inflammation goes hand-in-hand with free radical damage.

Dr. Lanksy developed a process creating potent pomegranate extracts combining fermented pomegranate juice, peel, leaves, flowers and seed. This combined antioxidant activity has a powerful synergy. Research demonstrated that the pomegranate extract's anti-inflammatory effect inhibited the inflammatory enzyme COX-2 by an impressive 31 to 44 percent.

Since estrogen dominance also exacerbates inflammatory conditions, this superior fermented pomegranate extract, in addition to its hormonal benefits also has a huge impact on reducing inflammation. This is *another huge plus* for women's hormonal health!

Pomegranate and Breast Health

The pomegranate is a paradoxical fruit. It has beneficial estrogenic properties as well as anti-estrogenic properties.

Dr. Lansky reported in *Breast Cancer Research and Treatment* that, according to published studies, his unique pomegranate extracts selectively inhibited or killed the growth of breast cancer cells in culture. His ongoing research has demonstrated the pomegranate extracts initiate eight different actions or mechanisms that can *prevent* breast cancer as well as *help in the treatment* of breast cancer:

- Suppresses breast cancer cells

- Interferes with cancer's growth cycle

- Inhibits products of hormones that stimulate cell growth

- Stops tumor cell invasion

- Initiates apoptosis, cell death

- Promotes cell differentiation

- Has anti-angiogenesis properties (stopping the growth of blood vessels to tumors)

- Acts as an aromatase inhibitor (stopping fats cells from making estrogen).

Pomegranate extracts are also able to effectively kill both estrogen positive and estrogen negative breast cancer cells.

A yet unpublished study conducted at Yale University found impressive results with the pomegranate extract with ovarian cancer. The study used the most virulent ovarian cancer lines, which had been resistant to all forms of treatment. The pomegranate extract was able to inhibit the cancer growth. In the future we may find that pomegranate extracts may have as much potential with ovarian cancer as well as it has with breast cancer. Other types of cancers have responded positively in studies using pomegranate extracts including prostate, stomach, lung cancers and leukemia.

According to Dr. Lansky, "Pomegranates are unique in that the hormonal combinations inherent in the fruit seem to be helpful both for the prevention and treatment of breast cancer. Pomegranates seem to replace needed estrogen often prescribed to protect postmenopausal women against heart disease and osteoporosis, while selectively destroying estrogen-dependent cancer cells."

Pomegranate for Vaginal Health

If there is one problem that is really the bane of a woman's existence, there's no doubt it would be vaginal dryness.

Vaginal dryness is a common problem for women during and after menopause, although inadequate vaginal lubrication can occur at any age. Symptoms of vaginal dryness include itching and stinging around the vaginal opening and in the lower third of the vagina. Vaginal dryness also makes intercourse uncomfortable which can certainly take its toll on relations as well!

A thin layer of moisture always coats your vaginal walls. Hormonal changes during your menstrual cycle and as you age affect the amount and consistency of this moisture. Most vaginal lubrication consists of clear fluid that seeps through the walls of the blood vessels encircling the vagina. When you're sexually aroused, more blood flows to your pelvic organs, creating more lubricating vaginal fluid. But the hormonal changes of menopause, childbirth and breast-feeding may disrupt this process.

Without adequate lubrication, the vaginal tissue becomes dry and thin. Besides painful intercourse, it can also lead to incontinence, bladder infections and pelvic floor problems. The only really effective solution has been the use of a vaginal estriol cream, which is not advised for women diagnosed with breast cancer or at high risk of breast cancer since. Even though it is a weaker form of estrogen, it can still increase estrogen levels.

This is where pomegranate can come to the rescue. Dr. Earl Surwit is a professor in the University of Arizona's College of Medicine who specializes in pelvic floor disorders and incontinence. He conducted a clinical study looking for alternatives to estrogen creams. Dr. Surwit investigated effects of a pomegranate lipid complex made from extracts of pomegranate fruit and pomegranate seed oil on vaginal dryness and pelvic floor disorders in older women. The results showed that the pomegranate lipid complex successfully restored vaginal lubrication and healthy vaginal tissue. It also had a positive effect on incontinence and helped to strengthen pelvic floor muscles. In every way, the pomegranate extract was as effective as estrogen creams without raising estrogen levels.

Vaginal Dryness Program

Here's the best natural program to address vaginal dryness. Use pomegranate seed oil, both topically, applying 2 - 4 drops daily to the vulva, and intravaginally. In addition, use a good pomegranate seed extract to help balance the entire hormonal system. Women who have been using the combination of pomegranate seed oil and the pomegranate extract to alleviate vaginal dryness, have reported an unexpected bonus. To their delight, they have experienced increased libido!

Pomegranate Seed Oil for Healthy, Glowing Skin

As it turns out pomegranate seed oil is also has many cosmetic benefits. Pomegranate seed oil has the ability to restore epithelial tissue, which means it helps repair and stimulates the regeneration of new skin cells. It can be used topically, directly on the hands and face to help stimulate new healthy cells for younger-looking skin, as well as orally, as a dietary supplement.

Pomegranate seed oil can help in the following ways:

❖ Nourishes and revitalizes your skin and your body

❖ Stalls the effects of aging while strengthening and supporting your immune system

❖ Soothes minor skin irritations as it smoothes away wrinkles

❖ Helps the body naturally restore moisture and health for those "intimate" needs

Back to the Future with Pomegranate Fruit

Ancient cultures have always regarded the pomegranate as a profound healing food. We've finally caught up to the Ancients. We finally know that the pomegranate fruit truly is a pharmacopoeia of health-promoting nutrients. It is evident that this amazing pomegranate fruit provides a cornucopia of health benefits for women.

The pomegranate plays a major role in helping women to regain and maintain their hormonal well-being throughout their lives. This beautiful fruit rightly deserves its place as a symbol of fertility, women's health, beauty and healing.

As the interest in the humble pomegranate continues to grow, ongoing research will no doubt reveal more of the many health-promoting secrets that Nature has hidden within the leathery red skin of this extraordinary fruit. Our 21st century knowledge will agree with the ancient wisdom: the pomegranate fruit is, indeed, the "Fruit of Life".

Chapter 8

The Antidote to Being Frazzled and Foggy

For millions of sleep-deprived Americans, a restful eight hours of shut-eye has become a rare luxury.

Sleep is the ultimate rejuvenation elixir. During deep sleep, brain activity that controls emotions, decision-making processes, and social interactions shuts down, allowing us to maintain optimal emotional and social functioning when we are awake.

A good night's sleep also plays a critical role in strengthening the body's immune defenses. One of the body's most powerful cancer fighters, called tumor necrosis factor, increases tenfold during a restful sleep. This is also the stage when cell growth and cell repair takes place.

In one study reported in *Psychosomatic Medicine*, volunteers were vaccinated against hepatitis A infection. When they had a good night's sleep afterwards, they showed a stronger immune response to the vaccine. The well-rested group displayed nearly twice the antibody level of the sleep-deprived group.

The quantity and quality of sleep impacts on many health problems. For example, insufficient sleep affects growth hormone secretion that is linked to obesity. It also impairs the body's ability to use the weight and appetite regulating hormones, insulin, leptin and gherlin.

Scientists have found increased blood levels of stress hormones in people with chronic insomnia, suggesting these people suffer from round-the-clock activation of the body's system for responding to stress. Insomniacs have increased production of the stress hormone cortisol, which not only prevents them from sleeping, but also leads to depression, high blood pressure, obesity, osteoporosis, and hormonal imbalances such as PMS, infertility, and menopausal symptoms.

In fact, the metabolic and endocrine changes resulting from a significant sleep debt mimic many of the hallmarks of aging.

However, reaching for that bottle of prescription sleeping pills or tranquilizers may not be your best choice. They not only shut down the brain, but prevent the mind from relaxing and recuperating, causing people to feel groggy or "out of it" upon waking. These medications also have numerous side effects and can be addictive.

L-theanine to the Rescue

There is something quite amazing about the Japanese people. Even though they live in one of the most stressed-out societies in the modern world, they are still considered extremely healthy people. In spite of the unrelenting demands and pressures of their culture, the Japanese people live longer than practically any other culture on the planet. What's more surprising is that have extremely low rates of obesity, heart disease, and breast cancer. What is the secret that allows them to not only survive their high-pressure life style but also actually thrive?

Green tea is the national drink of Japan and it has been so for hundreds of years. It is such an intrinsic part of Japanese life that the tea ceremony, an elaborate ritual for the preparation and serving of green tea has become an important cultural expression. This ancient ceremony embodies the essence of the healing benefits bestowed by green tea—the calming of the body, the stilling of the mind and the soothing of the soul.

Drinking tea has long been popular in Asian countries not the least for its many health benefits, including its calming influence on the mind and body. What makes green tea so special?

Taiyo International, a leading manufacturer of functional

foods, found this relaxation effect to be due to the presence of the amino acid L-theanine, found almost exclusively in tea. The purest source of l-theanine is called Suntheanine.

One of Suntheanine benefits is its ability to initiate an alpha brain wave pattern that signifies a relaxed physical and mental state without drowsiness or impaired motor skills. An alpha state also helps improve learning and concentration, strengthen the immune system, and alleviate stress-induced hormonal imbalances Suntheanine also increases levels of dopamine, another brain chemical with mood-enhancing effects.

A research study published in 2001 in *Alternative and Complementary Therapies* found an increased alpha brain wave pattern just 30 to 40 minutes after consuming 50 mg to 200 mg of a Suntheanine supplement.

Suntheanine's relaxation effect is caused by its ability to cross the blood-brain barrier, stimulating the formation of the neurotransmitter, GABA (gamma-aminobutyric acid). This neurotransmitter promotes a state of deep relaxation and calm, and at the same time increases sensations of pleasure. GABA is our body's own natural relaxant! By maintaining adequate levels of GABA, we are able to experience a sense of well being and inner peace, no matter what our stress levels may be!

A clinical trial at the National Institute of Mental Health in Japan involving 22 young men pointed to l-theanine's ability to promote quality sleep. When 200 mg of l-theanine was taken before bedtime, it enhanced the quality of actual sleep of all the participants. In fact, upon waking, all reported a significant absence of "feeling exhausted," and a reduced need for sleep. The study also indicated that l-theanine produced a notable improvement in sleep efficiency—an index of actual sleep time enjoyed between the time of falling asleep and waking. To add icing to the cake, test subjects reported a superior mental state prior to falling asleep and a decrease in nightmares.

The study confirmed that l-theanine improves the quality of sleep by allowing the mind to fully relax and recuperate. This is why the subjects did not report feeling groggy and felt refreshed and alert upon waking.

Suntheanine has many and varied proven health benefits. While not a sedative, Suntheanine is able to significantly improve the quality of sleep, so you wake up feeling truly rested and refreshed. In addition, it helps cells to better recognize foreign antigens and triggers the release of virus-destroying compounds in the cells. In addition, Suntheanine has proven itself as effective protection to the liver from the damaging effects of alcohol by increasing levels of the body's most potent antioxidant called glutathione.

A study published in the *Proceedings of the National Academy of Sciences* demonstrated that Suntheanine helps prepare the immune system to fight against foreign substances such as bacteria, viruses and fungi. Another human study out of Harvard University showed that blood cells of tea drinkers (tea contains L-theanine) reacted five times faster to germs than did those of coffee drinkers.

New research findings with an abundant amino acid in tea, indicate a protective effect against the cellular side effects that accompany chemotherapy and prevention of nerve cell degeneration.

A recent Suntheanine study should be especially good news for women. Taking 200 mg Suntheanine daily has been demonstrated to dramatically reduce the physical and emotional symptoms of PMS. Further more, it can uplift and enhance moods, making it a safe antidote to depression and anxiety.

Studies have shown that Suntheanine helps to:

❖ Improve learning and memory by regulating the levels of dopamine and serotonin. Alleviate normal symptoms of premenstrual stress (PMS). Irritability, nervousness, anxiety, and crying are just some of the symptoms that can be helped by daily use of Suntheanine for women suffering from PMS.

❖ Support the immune system by reducing stress. Stress can be very damaging to the immune system.

- ❖ Improve the overall quality of sleep by allowing the mind to fully relax and recuperate (when taken before bedtime)

- ❖ Promote a positive mood and alertness.

- ❖ Reduce anxiety and nervous tension.

- ❖ Improve the quality of sleep, reduce hyperactive behaviors and improve cognitive performance in children with ADHD.

Be sure to use only the purest form of Suntheanine by Taiyo, which has the safety and efficacy studies behind it, as well as the FDA confirmation on its safety.

The recommended amount of Suntheanine is 50-200 mg. It is also safe for children. Usually the calming effects are felt within 30 minutes and lasts from 8 to 12 hours.

Chapter 9

What's Up with this Weight Gain?

Like so many women, the mid-life middle spread seemed to have sneaked up on me. I knew I had just emerged from two years of major life changes with its accompanying stress. Well, really, to be totally honest, MAJOR STRESS! However, I was not at all prepared for my doctor's rather blunt comment.

Rather tactlessly he said. "What has happened to you? You look like you are six months pregnant."

Now I knew I had been carrying some extra cortisol-induced weight around the midriff, but I guess denial is a really wonderful thing. I really didn't think I looked that overweight. Stepping onto his scale really ripped the veil of illusion from my eyes!

For most women, weight gain is the bane of our existence. It is a culturally induce fat phobia. Aside from our vanity, extra-weight is a health hazard. In 2004 the U.S. Centers for Disease Control and Prevention (CDC) ranked obesity as the number one health threat facing America. More than 60 percent of women over the age of 20 fall into the overweight category. That's makes it 64.5 million of us! If we're talking obesity that means almost 35 million more are in that category.

Americans spend a lot of money on weight loss programs and diets.

$50 billion annually!

That's an awful lot of our hard earned cash!

Whether we like it or not, the older we get the less efficient our body becomes at detoxifying, maintaining a dynamic metabolism, balancing hormones and managing blood sugar. All of these issues can add to ever upward-creeping weight. Popular drugs also play their part. It is well acknowledged that HRT, anti-depressants, statins, and blood pressure medications list weight gain as side-effects!

I have not been immune from this obsession with body image. There were times when I have been thin. And then there were times when I have been fat. I dieted and fasted and cleansed and starved and exercised until I was blue in the face!

Over the years I cleaned up my nutritional regime. I basically ate a gluten-free, sugar-free, soda-free, processed-food free, organic food diet. I exercised (sometimes). I made the extra effort to manage my stress levels. I took my nutritional supplements. I balanced my hormones (naturally). I went to sleep at a decent hour (going to bed after 11 pm and getting less than 7 hours increases weight gain).

I thought I was doing everything right but my weight loss was stalled. I couldn't get it to budge. So, it's no wonder that my doctor's comment was such a blow to my self-image and my fruitless efforts!!!!

Enter the Ultimate Fat Loss and Body Resculpting Program

One day, a chance comment about a new kind of weight loss program changed my life. I was introduced to HCG, Human Chorionic Gonatrophin, an obscure hormone that I had never heard of before.

It seems that HCG plays a major role in our survival. I learned that although it is produced in every cell in our body, it is found in very high amounts during pregnancy. One of its jobs is to ensure the survival of the pregnant mother and fetus by signaling the hypothalamus to release stored fat to be used as fuel and nourishment. Under the command of HCG, these fats reserves will provide 1500-2000 calories a day of energy and nutrition.

However, it is important to emphasize that HCG is a hormone found naturally in both sexes. Its action is identical in men, women, and children, young and old alike.

Its message is simple—open the rusty hinges on those doors holding in long term storage fat.

What HCG does for a pregnant women, is what it can also do for the rest of us. This amazing hormone has become the key ingredient to one of the most successful permanent fat loss and resculpting programs ever created. We have Dr. A.T.W. Simeons to thank for that.

Dr. Simeons was an English medical doctor who discovered that HCG had a major impact on fat loss by regulating the hypothalamus. The main function of this master gland is homeostasis, or maintaining the body's status quo. Ultimately the hypothalamus can control every endocrine gland in the body. It also regulates other factors such as blood pressure, body temperature, fluid and electrolyte balance, and body weight.

The message that HCG gives the body is to release reserves of long-term stored fat. That's the ugly fat that we struggle so hard to rid ourselves of. It's the fat that is stored in our abdomen, thighs and hips. This is also the fat that accumulates as fat pads in our arms, knees, back and neck. For men, it's the fat that piles up in their abdomen, making them look several months pregnant.

The most frustrating thing about this variety of fat is that no amount of dieting will ever touch it. It is only accessible with HCG. The body seems to hold on to it for dear life as part of its survival strategy.

The first to go when we start the usual, run-of-the-mill diet is water, muscle and subcutaneous fat—the fat that gives shape to our face and fullness to our breasts. No wonder most diets result in saggy and toneless skin.

But HCG is totally different. It releases ONLY the long term stored fat, it actually helps the body to properly redistribute weight and regain firmness in the body. So on the HCG program you not only lose pounds, you lose inches! No sagging… no loose skin. In fact, it actually helps to tone your body.

And the most amazing thing is that Dr. Simeons discovered people were able to lose a pound of fat a day on average. While most weight loss programs recommend 1 or 2 pounds a week, the HCG program enables people to lose as much as a pound a day as well as eliminating inches!

An important aspect of this program is the discovery that the HCG program actually resets the body's metabolism. When the program is followed precisely, you are able to regain a healthy metabolism. This is key to making sure your weight will stay off. Yo-yoing can then become a thing of the past.

The Thyroid Is Not the Answer

I used to believe that the thyroid would help with fat loss. However, according to Dr. Simeons, that is not the case. In fact, the thyroid plays no part in releasing the fat that causes us to be overweight and obese.

This was quite a revelation to me!

Dr. Simeons writes:

When it was discovered that the thyroid gland controls the rate at which body-fuel is consumed, it was thought that by administering thyroid gland to obese patients their abnormal fat deposits could be burned up more rapidly.

This, too, proved to be entirely disappointing because as we now know, these abnormal deposits take no part in the body's energy-turnover—they are inaccessibly locked away.

Thyroid medication merely forces the body to consume its normal fat reserves, which are already depleted in obese patients, and then to break down structurally essential fat without touching the abnormal deposits. In this way a patient may be brought to the brink of starvation in spite of having a hundred pounds of fat to spare.

Thus any weight loss brought about by thyroid medication is always at the expense of fat of which the body is in dire need.

Dr. Simeons' Gift to an Overweighted World

Dr. Simeons' program was a major innovation for the approach to permanent weight loss. He established a successful clinic in Rome in the 1960's, which catered to the rich and famous. There are many clinics in Europe and South America that continue to use Dr. Simeons' program successfully.

The good news is that you no longer need to be a celebrity to afford the wonderful benefits of HCG.

While Dr. Simeons original program revolved around injections of HCG, there is now a more convenient and easy method to get the exact same results.

Are you skeptical of such a program? Well, I certainly was. The original program required a daily subcutaneous self-administered injection of HCG. There was no way I would do that.

But I then learned that there was another HCG option. This involved taking oral drops of an HCG homeopathic remedy daily. Homeopathy, a 200 year old healing approach, based on the emerging science of energy medicine that imprints the energy of a substance without using the actually physical substance. The body is literally able to read the information and create the desired outcome. In the case of homeopathic HCG, it has the exact same effect as the more unpleasant and expensive HCG hormone injections.

The best part is its absolute effectiveness and safety.

So, I decided to give it a try. Using the HCG homeopathic drops along with following Dr. Simeons' protocol of specific foods in specific amounts for a specific period of time I embarked on this experiment. The best part of all, this program requires no specific exercise routines nor expensive eating plans nor special dietary formulas.

Now for most of us, stepping onto a scale to weigh in is equivalent to an extreme masochistic act. However, on this HCG program, it was closer to a religious experience. I would step on the scale in the morning and literally discover that a pound of fat had literally dematerialized from my body every day.

But it wasn't only the fat. It was also the inches. My old clothes were literally falling off me. I wasn't hungry at all. My energy was off the charts. And before my very eyes I saw my body transforming. The midriff disappeared and my hips and thighs are the thinnest they have ever been since my 16th birthday! An accomplishment I never thought possible in this lifetime! And wonders of wonders—my muscle tone actually improved.

Unbelievable!

During this 23-day protocol, I lost 15 pounds and 2 dress sizes!

The most impressive part of this amazing program was that by resetting my hypothalamus and my metabolism, my weight has not varied more than a pound in several months. It appears that Dr. Simeons was right. By improving metabolic functioning on the HCG program, there is a greater likelihood that this new weight loss is here to stay.

Since venturing into the HCG world, I have assisted many of my patients and friends on this protocol. Every single one of them has been successful. Men seem to have a fat loss advantage over women; they are much bigger losers on this program. However, the good news is that everyone can be a big loser!

Not only did they loss pounds and inches, they have all gained health benefits—joint and knee aches and pains disappeared, blood sugar levels returned to normal, blood pressure was lowered, sleep improved, energy increased, skin tone rejuvenated and food cravings disappeared.

It's not often that a weight loss program can deliver such fabulous results. In fact, there is no weight loss program that I know of that can safely release long term fat reserves nor reset the hypothalamus for on-going weight maintenance.

Could the wonderful discovery of Dr. Simeons be the solution for the growing epidemic of the obesity epidemic with all of the accompanying chronic health problems?

I have no doubt that in our diet-crazed world of people desperately seeking help, this is truly is the ultimate fat loss and body resculpting program!

I have now developed an integrated program based on Dr. Simeons' work using a comprehensive homeopathic protocol. To learn more about it please visit my website: www.whatwomenmustknow.com.

Thank you Dr. Simeons for providing the answer to our weight loss prayers.

Chapter 10

Let Food Be Your Medicine

In a world plagued by ever-increasing chronic disease, it may be time to look to the past for answers and follow the wisdom of ancient healers. "Let your food be your medicine and your medicine your food" summed up one of the key principles espoused more than 2500 years ago by Hippocrates, the father of medicine. His golden rule highlighted the importance of good nutrition as the foundation for optimal well-being. Instead of the pharmacy shelves, could the elixir of good health actually be found in the wholesome nutrition of nutrient-dense foods?

Unfortunately, such wholesome foods are difficult to find these days. Modern agricultural practices have essentially destroyed the nutritional value of most of our commercially grown and commonly used foods. US Senate Document 264 stated that "Laboratory tests prove that the fruits, the vegetables, the grains, the eggs and even the milk and meats of today are not what they were a few generations ago…. and the foods no longer contain certain amounts of minerals and are starving us, no matter how much we eat." (This was published in 1936!)

It's a national tragedy to discover just how mineral deficient and deprived of nutrients our soils and thus, our foods, have become. When the processing of foods as well as chemical ingredients are added to the mix, real nutrition has all but disappeared from the American diet. Our plates may be full, but our bodies are literally starving for nutrition.

Our modern world is truly in desperate need of a nutrient dense, super-hero food!

The Return of the Super-Seed

The advanced Aztec civilization was renowned for their extraordinary health, amazing stamina, and impressive strength. Ancient manuscripts have revealed that as early as 3500 B.C., a tiny super-seed was the nutritional foundation of this vast and prosperous nation. The seed was known as Salvia hispanica L, a member of the mint family.

The Aztecs consumed these seeds in a variety of ways. They were eaten alone, mixed with other seed crops, made into a beverage, ground into flour, included in medicines, and pressed for oil.

For more than 500 years, all knowledge of this seed became lost in the mists of time after the Conquistadors destroyed its cultivation. Fortunately, in 1991 two Argentinian brothers rediscovered Salvia Hispanica L. Through meticulous traditional plant breeding to maximize its nutritional benefits, they developed an extraordinary variety, called Salba with an even more superior nutrient composition than the ancient seed.

A World of Nutrition in A Tiny Seed

Modern science has recently discovered what the Aztecs always knew; this humble grayish-white seed contains a treasure trove of phenomenal nutrition. Recent research into Salba's exceptional nutritional value has hailed it as nature's most nutrient dense super-seed.

The true miracle of Salba's exceptional nutritional profile was discovered from research conducted by Vladimir Vuksan, a Professor of Endocrinology at University of Toronto. Dr. Vuksan is one of the world's experts renowned for developing novel alternative therapies for obesity, diabetes and heart disease.

Dr. Vuksan found that as a functional food, this gluten-free seed achieved two world firsts.

It's first claim to fame was that it had the highest known whole food source of Omega-3 Fatty Acids.

Omega-3 Fatty Acids are crucial for good health; regulating heart rate, blood pressure, blood clotting, fertility, immune support, improving mental health and reducing body inflammation. The National Institute of Health believes that most people need to at least double or triple their daily intake of Omega-3's Fatty Acids.

This is where Salba comes to the rescue. Just two tablespoons (15 grams) offers more than 3000 mg of Omega-3 Fatty Acids (in an optimal Omega-3 to Omega-6 ratio), supplying more than 100 percent of the recommended daily intake.

If that wasn't enough to make a superstar out of Salba, it has the highest dietary fiber content of any food, providing more than 5 grams in just 2 tablespoons (30 percent of your daily requirement). The soluble and insoluble fiber is in perfect balance. It not only increases bulk and transit time and alleviates constipation, but also helps to maintain both healthy blood glucose and blood cholesterol levels.

With such high fiber content, Salba provides superior ammunition in the battle of the bulge! Salba has the ability to absorb 14 times its weight in water. When added to meals it becomes a bulking agent, ensuring slower digestion and a slower rise in blood sugar. Salba's fiber content, thus, stabilizes blood sugar levels, along with creating a sense of fullness.

When made into a gel by soaking the seeds in water, Salba was also able to increase cellular hydration and electrolyte balance.

When measuring nutrients gram for gram, Salba has six times more calcium than whole milk, three times more iron than spinach, the potassium content of $1\frac{1}{2}$ large bananas, as much vitamin C as seven oranges, fifteen times more magnesium than broccoli, and three times the antioxidant capacity of blueberries. Adding to this long list, Salba contains naturally occurring folate, B vitamins, zinc, selenium, and vitamin A. Salba also has more bioavailable and complete protein than soy.

What's amazing is that such a high-powered food has less that 1/2 gm. net carbohydrate per serving.

Women's Health and Salba

Getting an adequate intake of omega-3's is vital for many women's health issues. First of all it, plays a major role in reducing inflammation in the body. Inflammation is now understood to play a major role in chronic illnesses such a diabetes, cardiovascular disease and cancer. Inflammation is also a factor in many women's hormonal issues such as endometriosis, fibroids, ovarian cysts, PMS and fibrocystic breasts.

The balance of omega-6 to omega-3 oils is critical to the proper metabolism of prostaglandins. LA and ALA can be converted to prostaglandins which are important for the regulation of inflammation, pain, blood pressure, fluid balance, blood clotting, steroid production and hormone synthesis, heart, kidney and gut function, and nerve function.

Breast health is also dependent on these health fats. Studies have shown that eating a high omega-3 fatty acid diet reduces your risk of breast cancer. If a woman has already been diagnosed, then omega-3's will help fight the disease. There are 4 ways that omega-3's help: they decrease the strength of estrogen in the breast tissue, reduce chronic inflammation, contribute to the shrinkage of breast tumors and prevent tumors from spreading. Women with the highest amount of omega-3 fatty acids in their bodies, have a 500 percent lower incidence of metastasis compared to women with the lowest levels of omega-3's.

Salba's high fiber content is important for hormone balance. Insoluble fiber helps to decrease estrogen overload by binding to the extra estrogen in the digestive tract. This extra estrogen is later eliminated from the body through the feces. Since extra estrogen, also known as estrogen dominance, is a major cause of just about every kind of hormonal issue, ensuring adequate fiber intake is a necessary strategy for healthy hormones.

A healthy endocrine system requires an abundance of minerals and vitamins. It is no secret that most of us are seriously depleted in these key nutrients. That's another reason why Salba's nutrient density is so beneficial for women of all ages.

There is one further health bonus; Salba is gluten-free. This makes it an ideal food for those with wheat and/or gluten sen-sitivities. Sub-clinical, or hidden, gluten intolerance is a health problem at epidemic proportions in certain populations in the United States and remains largely unrecognized by conventional medicine. Sub-clinical gluten intolerance creates a significant stress on the immune system and can lead to a compromised immune system. It also creates inflammation in the digestive tract. There is also a link between gluten intolerance and hypo-thyroid conditions, especially Hashimoto's Thyroiditis, a com-mon autoimmune condition of the thyroid. Gluten-free foods are a pre-requisite for women seeking hormonal balance.

The Healing Power for Diabetes and Metabolic Syndrome

Intrigued by Salba's superior nutrient composition, Dr. Vuksan conducted clinical studies using Type 2 Diabetic patients and healthy individuals. He made the following observations:

- ❖ Salba reduced after meal blood glucose and plasma insulin levels, thus improving the Glycemic Index of any food consumed with Salba

- ❖ C-Reactive protein, a marker for low grade body in-flammation was significantly lowered (40 percent)

- ❖ Salba significantly lowered systolic blood pressure

- ❖ Salba significantly decreased coagulation (blood thinning) by 30 percent

- ❖ No adverse effect was noted on glycemic control or blood lipids as previously seen with high doses of Omega-3 Fatty Acids

"These were huge discoveries rarely seen in medical litera-ture, even with the "Reduction of eight units of the systolic blood pressure represents a major health improvement; there aren't many studies showing this effect. We measured the body inflammation, the so-called C-reactive protein, which has been discovered as a major risk factor for heart disease, which seems to be even more important than cholesterol. A reduction of CRP, of about 32 percent in patients with Type 2 Diabetes who were heavily medicated and well controlled is not commonly seen in medical literature."

These studies were irrefutable evidence that consumption of Salba results in a simultaneous reduction of blood pressure, body inflammation and blood clotting, while balancing after-meal blood sugar.

It's no wonder why Dr. Vuksan is so excited about the results. "Due to Salba's extremely high Omega-3 Fatty Acids and its nutrient rich composition and results, Salba creates exceptional possibilities for the improvement of human health and nutrition. To my knowledge, nothing else in the field of nutrition has come close to matching these exceptional results. Salba can be considered an almost perfect functional food."

A World of Nutrition for Us All

So, who can benefit from eating Salba? With such a complete world of nutrition packed in to every little seed, it is obvious that everyone can benefit! It is an ideal food for weight loss, balancing hormones, and improving sports performance. In addition, Salba provides nutrition for children and the elderly. It is an excellent food for vegetarians and vegans allowing them to attain their protein and essential fatty acid needs. By balancing blood sugar levels as well as reducing inflammation, Salba is ideal for preventing or treating heart disease and diabetes.

With a growing focus on the need to improve children's health, Salba provides a great nutritional boost. It is already being incorporated as a "stealth health grain" in some school lunch programs.

The recommended daily serving of Salba for an adult is 2 tablespoons and children can take up to one tablespoon daily.

Salba's super star nutritional status is equally matched by its extraordinary versatility. It can be eaten either in its whole seed form or can be ground into flour using a simple home coffee grinder. Salba can be added to yogurt, cereal, salads, beverages, casseroles, breads, and cakes. It can also be used to thicken soups, stews, or sauces. Salba's neutral flavor makes is an ideal addition to just about any recipe. Be sure to look for a brand new generation of Salba-fortified healthy snack foods such as tortilla chips, breads, cookies, muffins, beverages, salsa, etc.

The seeds of the past have returned to the present to provide a promise for a healthier future.

Salba Banana Coconut Muffins

The best gluten-free, sugar-free, low-carb, nutrient-dense muffins!

2 Tbs. coconut oil
3 room-temperature eggs
1/3 cup mashed banana (1 small ripe banana)
1 tsp. alcohol-free vanilla flavor (such as Frontier Herbs) or vanilla extract
1/4 tsp. salt
1/4 cup coconut flour
2 Tbs. salba seeds
1/4 tsp. baking powder
1/2 tsp. ground cinnamon
1 Tbs. shredded coconut
2 Tbs. raisins or dried cranberries (optional)

Preheat oven to 400°F. Mix together oil, eggs, banana, vanilla, and salt.

Add coconut flour, salba, baking powder, cinnamon, and shredded coconut, and whisk together until smooth.

Fold in raisins or cranberries.

Pour into muffin cups greased with coconut oil.

Bake 15 minutes or until toothpick inserted in center of muffins comes out clean. Cool on wire rack.

Chapter 11

Super Charge Your Immune System

Have you ever wondered why an infant can eat food directly off a dirty floor and still stay healthy? Or, why you can be surrounded by a crowd of sneezing, coughing, sniffling people and still successfully weather the viral onslaught?

We have one of the miracles of our human body to thank for our impressive resilience—our amazingly intricate and intelligent immune system.

Every second of every day it is waging a silent war against billions of harmful bacteria, viruses, pathogens, fungi and parasites. Without a vigorous and effective immune system, our health, and, in fact, our lives would be in serious jeopardy.

Our ability to recover from any kind of acute as well as chronic illness necessitates a functioning and responsive immune system. When our immune system is strong, we are well. However, when it falters or fails, we are vulnerable to many illnesses.

Modern life poses many challenges to our immunity. Stress, pollution, nutritional deficiencies, allergens, surgery, insufficient sleep, electromagnetic radiation, free radicals, medications and even aging contribute to a weakened immune system.

Symptoms of comprised immunity include allergies, frequent colds and flu, sinus, ear, throat, skin, urinary tract, endometriosis and vaginal infections. Slow healing wounds, chronic fatigue, candidiasis, and of course degenerative diseases such as cancer, HIV, and autoimmune conditions are also due to a weakened immune state.

With so many daily assaults, it is no surprise that over half of all Americans suffer from a compromised immune system.

Keeping our immune system fighting fit must become a high priority for us all.

Our Intelligent Immune System

Like a modern army, our immunity entails a highly evolved and astonishingly sophisticated defense system with complex communications that provide specific instructions to highly specialized, well-trained soldiers. Together this integrated system can recognize foreign invaders or antigens and react against them appropriately.

Two types of immunity exist in our bodies: innate and adaptive. Innate immunity is present at birth and provides an initial barrier against microorganisms. Adaptive immunity is acquired later in life, such as after fighting off an infection: Adaptive immunity "remembers" these invaders and adapts to recognize and ward them off again should they recur at a future time.

Our immunity depends on a network of organs that includes lymph nodes, bone marrow, spleen, thymus gland, tonsils and adenoids, the appendix, and clumps of lymphoid tissue in the small intestine known as Peyer's patches. They are concerned with the growth, development, and deployment of lymphocytes, the white cells that are key operatives of the immune system

The adult body contains over a trillion lymphocytes that can be divided into different groups known as T cells, B cells and Natural Killer cells (NT cells)

B cells originate in the bone marrow and produce antibodies to kill antigens (any kind of foreign particle entering the body). T cells originate in the bone marrow but are matured and "educated" in the thymus. They are trained to detect and kill specific antigens as well as releasing chemicals known as cytokines. These are information molecules that communicate with and direct all the immune cells. Without them the immune system is deaf, dumb and blind.

NK cells are the body's first line of defense. They are the first to recognize an invader and rush to attack without prior sensitization. NK cells especially target host cells that have become cancerous as well as cells infected with viruses. Their weapon is a lethal chemical injected into the invaders killing them within minutes. This drama is reenacted 10,000 times every day as cancer cells are formed and destroyed in a healthy person's body. If this activity stops or slows down, the cancer cells are free to grow and become a clinical case of cancer.

The absolute number of NK cells gives little indication of the efficiency of immune function. Instead, it is the activity of the NK cells (how aggressive they are in recognizing and binding to tumor cells) that is important. People with low NK cells are more likely to experience auto-immune diseases, chronic fatigue, immune dysfunction, infections (e.g. Lyme Disease, Herpes Virus and Influenza Virus) and cancer. One of the effects of aging is the reduced activity of NK cells.

PeakImmune4 – A Biological Response Modulator to the Rescue

In the search for an effective and non-toxic immune-modulator, we need look no further than to a natural solution, in the form of a unique food supplement called PeakImmune4.

PeakImmune4 was developed in 1992 by Daiwa Pharmaceutical in Japan, after it was proven that polysaccharides from the fibrous part of rice bran extract when broken down by enzymes from shiitake mushrooms could actually strengthen the immune system. Unlike dietary fiber laxative products that do not enter the bloodstream, this unique fiber has been broken down so it can pass into the blood stream and reach the cells of the immune system.

The resulting compound, a patented arabinoxylan compound, has since been clinically shown to dramatically increase the activity of NK cells in patients with cancer (including difficult to treat blood cancers such as leukemia and multiple myelomas), immune compromised illnesses, and viral and autoimmune diseases.

When taken as a food supplement, PeakImmune4 increases the activity of the body's white blood cells—particularly T and B cell and especially Natural Killer (NK) cell function. With daily supplementation, NK cell activity is increased by more than 300 percent, B-cell activity by more than 250 percent and T cell activity by 200 percent "without overstimulating the immune system."

In addition, PeakImmune4 is able to keep white cell levels up from the immunosuppressive effects of chemotherapy and radiotherapy. PeakImmune4 is helpful in reducing the debilitating side effects of chemotherapy such as tiredness, nausea and weight loss while increasing the treatment's effectiveness.

More recent research has shown that PeakImmune4 also seems to lower the inflammatory responses of the immune system. As inflammation promotes the cancer process, reducing inflammation may be an important means of protection against cancer.

Research also shows that PeakImmune4 can inhibit replication of the HIV virus without damaging healthy cells, and studies have suggested that it may also be useful in the treatment of hepatitis C.

The really good news is that, unlike other immunomodulators, PeakImmune4 is completely non-toxic.

A Life Saving Supplement

PeakImmune4 has helped thousands of people around the world not only regain their lives but also to improve their quality of life.

Barbara's personal odyssey with a life threatening cancer is an inspiring example of the power of PeakImmune4. Eight years ago she was shocked when diagnosed with a rare aggressive thyroid cancer, which had spread into her chest. In a

12 hour life or death surgery, she had her thyroid removed as well as her chest tumors. Two months later the tumor grew back. Once again she had to make another life or decision. Would she agree to 33 radiation treatments?

Terrified of the prospect of radiation as well as a rapidly growing cancer, she prayed for a miracle. Her prayers were answered when she saw a magazine article about PeakImmune4.

She took the therapeutic dose of 3 gms daily before starting radiation and every day since then. Eight years later, she has defied her doctor's predictions and all the odds. Her NK cells remain high; her tumors have shrunk and are stable. Most importantly, she feels great.

Recently, a 3-month case study was conducted with five people with various stages of cancer and 2 observational individuals who were terminal. The purpose of the observational study was to learn more about effectiveness of PeakImmune4 on an array of factors, which may favorably impact human health and longevity.

The director of the study, Carol Blair, CN reports on the outcome for two of the participants. One was a 39 year old female at high risk of colon cancer with Familial Adenomatous Polyposis, a genetic condition in which numerous polyps form mainly in the large intestines. At end of the study, the examination showed the presence of only tiny clusters instead of large polyps. She was cleared for 1 year instead of a check-up every 3 months. .

The other participant was a 49 year old man with multiple tumors of the endocrine glands. At time of the study, he had tumors in the pancreas with metastases to the liver. While taking PeakImmune4 no new tumors developed. When entering the study he was depressed and felt quite hopeless. By the end of the study he experienced improved energy and felt that "Life is worth living again. I don't know what I would do without PeakImmune4."

Carol Blair commented about the study's outcome. "As a result of our study, I was impressed with the overall health benefits of PeakImmune4. Not only did the participants experience increased NK cell activity as measured on their blood tests, but they also suffered from fewer colds and influenzas that were going around at that time. Most of them also reported increased energy. The 2 terminal patients had a longer life than was expected by their oncologists and a better quality of life. All of the others measured higher NK cells."

A Strong Immune System is Your Best Health Insurance

In addition to an impressive increase in NK cell activity, PeakImmune4 also has other immune-boosting effects: it increases levels of interferon, a compound produced by the body that inhibits the replication of viruses; it increases the formation of Tumor Necrosis Factors, a group of proteins that help destroy cancer cells, and it increases the activity of T-cells and B-cells.

PeakImmune4 has also been used to treat hepatitis B and C. People in "high risk" categories for disease can benefit from using PeakImmune4 preventively. These include people who smoke and drink, people exposed to toxic chemicals, people born with immune deficiencies, and members of families with a strong history of cancer.

Since persistently depressed NK cell activity was found in 14 percent of "healthy" young adults, it is becoming apparent that PeakImmune4 offers the immune boosting ability that can benefit people of all ages.

Since we live in a world that severely taxes our immunity, without a doubt, our best health insurance is a powerful immune system.

Chapter 12

Glutathione – The Miracle Molecule for Longevity

Recent statistics have good news for us. Centenarians are the fastest growing age group in America. What's the secret to a long and healthy life? And, what can you do right now to ensure that you will one day take your place in the ranks of vibrant 100 year olds?

The answer can very well be found in the presence of a small but potent molecule made in every cell of your body called glutathione. While glutathione may not have the same notoriety as other more high profile nutrients such as vitamin C and E, it certainly is a miracle molecule.

Glutathione levels of 41 centenarians between the ages of 100-105 years old were compared with those people between 60-79 years old. They found that the mean glutathione activity was significantly higher in centenarians than in the group of younger elderly subjects, and that centenarians with the best functional capacity tended to have the highest glutathione activity.

The study concluded that high glutathione levels are associated with increased survival.

In a later study, glutathione levels were evaluated in 87 women in excellent physical and mental health, ranging in age from 60 to 103. The scientists found that all women had very high blood glutathione levels. They followed these women for five years, and concluded "high blood glutathione concentrations … are characteristic of long-lived women."

The Life-Extending Master Antioxidant

Glutathione (GSH) is a tripeptide molecule composed of three amino acids: glutamic acid, cysteine and glycine. It is one of the main nonprotein antioxidants that exists within each cell, and has been referred to as the body's "master antioxidant." It rules the body's cells and is abundant in cytoplasm, nuclei and the mitochondria.

Although discovered in 1888, the initial research on glutathione deficiency was conducted in the 1920's and 1930's and concentrated on the eye, particularly the lens. It is well known that macula degeneration is related to low levels of glutathione. By the 1980's, researchers realized that glutathione was a major player in all aspects of good health and disease prevention.

Without adequate glutathione levels, each cell would eventually disintegrate from massive free radical damage, your body would have little resistance to metabolic waste products and your liver would be severely compromised from the eventual accumulation of toxins. Our cells would also be defenseless against the many bacteria, viruses and many of the carcinogens that pose a health threat.

For the past three decades, researchers have been investigating the role of antioxidants for the maintenance of good health as well as for the prevention and treatment of oxidative stress-induced diseases.

The better known antioxidants such as vitamin A, vitamin E and selenium must be obtained from the diet. However, glutathione is considered the master antioxidant because all other antioxidants depend upon its presence to function properly. For example, it is essential in regenerating oxidized forms of vitamins C and E by recirculating them back into antioxidant function. Normally once these antioxidant vitamins scavenge free radicals, they can become oxidized themselves and attack the healthy cells. This is known as pro-oxidation. Glutathione easily restores them to their reduced form so they can resume the free radical scavenging activity again.

When the glutathione systems are functioning effectively,

the use of antioxidants maximizes their effectiveness in the treatment and prevention of degenerative diseases associated with oxidative stress. This includes arthritis, cancer, cardiovascular diseases, diabetes and macular degeneration

Glutathione performs important jobs in the body which includes protecting cells against the destructive effects of free radicals; detoxifying external substances such as drugs, environmental pollutants and carcinogens; maintaining cell membrane stability; regulating protein and DNA biosynthesis and cell growth; enhancing immunologic function through its influence on lymphocytes; prostaglandin synthesis; and amino acid transport.

Since it is involved in so many critical functions, glutathione impacts all levels of the body's physiological functioning.

It is believed that glutathione has the potential to treat and prevent hundreds of diseases. When you consider the role that glutathione plays in the basic wellness of cells, the primary living building blocks in our body, you can appreciate why maintaining glutathione levels is critical for optimal wellbeing.

Essential Support of Immunity and Detoxification

In addition to its role as a powerful antioxidant, glutathione also serves as an immune system enhancer and a detoxifier.

As an immune system enhancer, glutathione is needed for the proper functioning, and in particular the creation and maintenance, of T-cells a type of lymphocytes, the body's frontline defense against infection.

Glutathione plays a central role in the proper function of the white blood cells. Dr. Gustavo Bounous, a glutathione expert, says, "The limiting factor in the proper activity of our lymphocytes (the white blood cells) is the availability of glutathione." The healthy growth and activity of the white blood cells depends upon high levels of intracellular glutathione.

In people with immune deficiency, glutathione levels fall well below the normal levels in blood and immune cells. Restoring glutathione levels to those found in healthy people has benefited immune deficient patients. Studies have suggested that, an increase in the glutathione level in the body can help patients with HIV (AIDS) to improve their survival.

In a toxic world, survival literally depends on the body's ability to adequately detoxify the tens of thousands of chemicals that inhaled, ingested, and absorbed into the body. Glutathione also comes to our rescue as a major detoxifier. The level of glutathione in the liver is critically linked to the liver's capacity to detoxify. This means that the higher the glutathione content, the greater the liver's capacity to detoxify harmful chemicals.

Glutathione is able to bind to organic toxins, as well as heavy metals, solvents and pesticides, and transform them into a form that can be excreted in urine or bile.

Glutathione's Role in Cancer Prevention

Columbia University School of Public Health, estimated that 95 percent of cancer is caused by diet and environmental toxicity. It is evident that in order to prevent cancer, it is imperative to protect the body from this onslaught of toxins.

Dr. Dean Jones PhD, Director of Nutritional Health Sciences at Emory University and glutathione expert states, "The role of glutathione that has probably received the most attention in the past 50 years is the function of glutathione as an anti-carcinogen. Glutathione is used to counter reactive chemicals that would otherwise cause mutations in the DNA and cause cancer. A little over 50 years ago it was recognized that many chemicals we are exposed to are activated in the body to reactive chemicals, the most central way that the body gets rid of these is by reacting these with glutathione. Glutathione is the most anticarcinogenic chemical we have in our body."

Most people do not inherit "cancer genes" but rather they have a genetic weakness in their detoxification system. Glutathione is an extremely important part of the detoxification system, and thus of our defenses against cancer.

The Miracle Molecule

As a powerful free radical scavenger, immune enhancer and detoxifier, glutathione has shown to be effective in the following conditions: autism, cardiovascular disease, autoimmune diseases, asthma, diabetes, lung disease, Parkinson's' disease, gastrointestinal inflammation and Crohn's disease, hepatitis, chronic fatigue syndrome, neuro-degenerative diseases such as MS (Multiple Sclerosis), ALS (Lou Gehrig's Disease), Alzheimer's and Parkinson's and degenerative eye conditions such as cataracts and macular degeneration.

Medical science is still ascertaining all the critical roles played by glutathione in disease resistance and general good health.

Staying healthy as well as recovering one's health requires maintaining high levels of glutathione. The older we get the more our levels of glutathione decline, especially after the age of 45. Therefore, shoring up your glutathione reserves is crucial.

Who needs to increase glutathione levels? If you have been diagnosed with a chronic illness, are in pain, have autism, are under stress, have digestive problems, have a weakened immune system, eat lots processed foods, engage in strenuous exercise, are overweight and feel fatigued, glutathione will be a real boost to your wellbeing.

And, if you are committed to staying healthy and energetic, then a successful anti-aging program necessitates maintaining high glutathione levels.

Increasing Glutathione Levels

When it comes to understanding the importance of glutathione, John P. Richie, Jr., Ph.D., professor at Penn State University School of Medicine is a world expert on the subject. He has been researching glutathione for over 25 years including its role in protecting against oxidative damage during aging and the development of cancer at numerous sites.

His research confirms the following findings. Numerous studies have supported the use of oral glutathione even though increases in glutathione levels may not be apparent in all tissues. For example, orally administered glutathione is not generally accompanied by an increase glutathione levels in the liver, which is the main storehouse and exporter of glutathione in the body. However, this lack of affect in the liver is not likely due to a lack of bioavailability. Research conducted by Dr. Richie and others clearly demonstrate the effectiveness of oral glutathione at enhancing the glutathione content of other critical tissues and protecting against a variety of important disease processes.

The very best way to ensure adequate glutathione levels is to provide the body with the key building blocks of glutathione.

There are two clinically proven products that increase intracellular glutathione. One effective product is called Setria® Glutathione manufactured by Kyowa Hakko U.S.A., Inc. It is a tripeptide composed of the glutathione precursors, glutamic acid, cysteine and glycine. Setria® Glutathione is an oral L-glutathione supplement manufactured using a proprietary fermentation process. Setria® Glutathione is a key ingredient found in many glutathione-promoting products.

A clinically proven product that increases intracellular glutathione is called MaxGXL developed by Robert Keller MD, MS, FACP, a renown cancer and AIDS researcher and clinician specializing in the fields of Internal Medicine, Immunology and Hematology. Dr. Keller has also been named as one of the worlds 2,000 Outstanding Scientists of the 21st Century, and has served on the scientific review panels for the National Institutes of Health and the Veterans Affairs.

MaxGXL provides the required nutrients needed to promote the body's own ability to manufacture and absorb glutathione. After years of research and development, Dr. Keller created MaxGXL, a product containing the necessary components of glutathione that, when absorbed into the body, stimulate the body's own production of glutathione in every cell of the body. MaxGXL also aids in liver support, thus helping the liver to function as the main production site and storehouse for glutathione. Since glutathione levels are lowest in the mornings, it is best to use all glutathione supplements early in the day.

Glutathione levels can also be increased in several other ways. Moderate, prolonged physical exercise increases glutathione and its related enzyme levels in the blood and skeletal muscles.

In addition, many vitamins and nutritional supplements are Glutathione boosters: lipoic acid, pines bark extract (pycnogenol), melatonin, bilberry, grape extract, vitamin C, whey protein, and turmeric have all been shown to elevate glutathione.

Glutathione is found primarily in fresh whole foods: raw fruits and vegetables, raw meats and fresh milk (unfortunately even milk storage reduces the glutathione level). Some of the foods that are high in glutathione include cruciferous vegetables, such as cauliflower, broccoli, cabbage, kale, and Brussels sprouts. But don't expect to find any glutathione in a junk food diet. It is non-existent in cereals, canned and processed foods, and cured meats.

While glutathione has a very long list of impressive benefits, its fundamental role is to improve, if not maximize, the function of every cell in every organ of your body. There are very few other factors, which are as predictive of our life expectancy as well as our levels of cellular glutathione.

So if you really want to be around to celebrate your 100th birthday, there's no time like the present to start revving up those glutathione levels!

Chapter 13

Drugs on Tap

Have you ever wondered what happens to the hundreds of millions of prescription drugs and over-the-counter medications that Americans swallow every day? Probably not. So, here's something to ponder as you're sipping your morning coffee or relaxing in your aromatherapy bath. Up to 90 percent of every drug that a person puts into his body is either eliminated unchanged or broken down into an active metabolite before being excreted down the toilet and into the sewage system where it finds its way into the water supplies. But then there's one more step to this chain of events, this drug ultimately returns to its source via the water faucet.

It is estimated that there are 129 widely used drugs in municipal waste water systems nationwide. They include antibiotics, antacids, antidepressants, birth control pills, hormone replacement therapy (estrogen and progestins), seizure medication, cancer treatments, painkillers, tranquilizers, cholesterol lowering compounds, caffeine and nicotine, to name just a few.

According to the U.S. Environmental Protection Agency, "the amount of pharmaceuticals and personal care products entering the environment annually is about equal to the amount of pesticides used each year."

This collection of chemical compounds is officially known as Pharmaceuticals and Personal Care Pollutants (PPCPs). They consist of a very broad and diverse assortment of thousands of chemical substances that Americans use on a daily basis. Little if any thought is given to the consequence as staggering quantities of these chemicals are washed down the sink, flushed down the toilet as human waste, or rinsed from our bodies into shower drains to be released into the environment.

Many pharmaceutical and personal care products have persistent chemicals and compounds that remain biologically active after they leave the body or are disposed into land fills and water systems. Hospitals, doctor's offices, veterinary clinics, farms, ranches and average homes are continual sources of PPCPs. It's a sobering thought to realize that each one of us, however unwittingly, is contributing to the PPCP's toxic load permeating our water systems.

PPCPs also find their way into the water from unused medications flushed down the toilet, through failing septic systems or discharged from wastewater treatment plants. Even though PPCPs are pervasive, very little research has been conducted about the potential effects of this low-level, long-term exposure to combinations of chemicals on human and aquatic life.

What does this mean for the environment? Many chemicals are designed to profoundly affect humans' physiology. Unlike pesticides, these drugs—as well as shampoos, sunscreens and other personal care products rushing down the drain—aren't examined for their effect on the environment before they're placed on the market. This is surprising especially since certain pharmaceuticals are designed to modulate endocrine and immune systems. Hence, they have obvious potential as endocrine disruptors in the environment.

Would You Like Birth Control Pills With Your Coffee?

Synthetic estrogen hormones are taken by millions of women for birth control and hormonal replacement therapies as well as prescribed to men for treatment of prostate cancer. Both natural and synthetic estrogens enter sewage treatment plants in large quantities; so do estrogen-mimicking chemicals from degradation of surfactants and plasticizers. Do these hormones interfere with vulnerable hormonal receptors in living creatures?

Results from a Canadian study provided concrete evidence of just what exposure to these chemicals portends. For three years, Canadian scientists added birth control pills to a remote Ontario Lake to measure its impact. The results: All male fish in the lake—from tiny tadpoles to large trout—were "feminized," meaning they had egg proteins growing abnormally in their bodies. Feminized male fish are now being found in rivers and streams throughout the world.

In river otters, frogs and other aquatic life populations, the effect is the same—the presence of female hormones is making the male species less male—much less male. Washington state scientists have found that synthetic estrogen can drastically reduce the fertility of male rainbow trout.

Some of the known potential impacts on organisms include delayed development in fish, delayed metamorphosis in frogs and a variety of reactions, including altered behavior and reproduction.

Evidence is already mounting on the impact to humans. One study found that rural men exposed to certain pesticides that act like estrogen had lower sperm counts. Could estrogen-laced water contribute to sharply falling human sperm counts? In Europe, researchers have tied a decline in male sperm count to levels of estrogenic hormones in the environment. What about the rising numbers of breast and uterine cancers, early puberty and hypospadias, a birth defect of the urethra and penis, from exposure to estrogenic compounds? It is not difficult to imagine how unnatural exposure to potent estrogen hormones, as well as estrogen mimics, could be a part of these growing trends to the hormonal health of both adults and children.

Antibiotics—Too Much of A Good Thing

Detection of antibiotics in drinking water is of particular concern because the presence of these chemicals in the environment may lead to the development of resistant bacterial strains, thus diminishing the therapeutic effectiveness of antibiotics.

Meanwhile, thousands of pounds of triclosan (the active ingredient in antibacterial soaps, deodorants, sponges and household cleaners) are also going down the drain into our waterways. Triclosan contributes to the resistance problem because it is a broad-spectrum antimicrobial agent, killing all bacteria on the body and household surfaces, even the beneficial kind. That, in turn, creates an environment where the superbugs can flourish.

Due to a germ phobia public, the use of antibacterial products is steadily growing. Too bad. Not only are they dangerous to the environment but they are also unnecessary and ineffective. According to the Center for Science in the Public Interest's project on antibiotic resistance, "The use of these products has never been shown to be superior, to my knowledge, to regular soap and water."

Just Drink Your Prozac and Call Me in the Morning

An estimated 164 million prescriptions for antidepressants were dispensed to 27 million Americans in 2005. That's a lot of happy pills. The most popular kind is the selective serotonin reuptake inhibitors (SSRIs), which include Prozac, Zoloft, Luvox and Paxil.

Researchers at Baylor University have found in Texas traces of Prozac and other antidepressants in the livers, muscles and brains of bluegill fish, along with traces in people who don't take Prozac but do eat fish.

In August 2004, major headlines in Britain announced that Prozac was found in U.K. drinking water. Environmentalists have described the situation as "hidden mass medication of the unsuspecting public." Since the U.K., like the U.S., has no monitoring of levels of Prozac or other PPCPs, a serious public health crisis is brewing. In the U.K. there has been a 166 percent increase in antidepressant prescriptions since 1991—up to 24 million prescriptions a year.

No one really knows what might be the effect when whole populations, including pregnant women and children, are getting traces of these drugs through their water supplies. It is known, however, that there can be serious side effects including depression, insomnia, hallucinations, self-mutilating behavior and violence.

Now that the problem of PPCPs has been clearly identified, the tricky part is what to do about it. To begin with, whenever possible choose nontoxic personal care products. They're better for your body and the environment. Consider investigating natural therapies instead of relying on pharmaceutical drugs. Use the political process and make your feelings known on a local, state and national level as well as supporting environmental organizations.

The day may come when pharmaceutical companies will take responsibility for the life cycle of their products; the EPA and FDA will enact protective regulations for PPCPs; and new sewage treatment technologies will be developed and installed. But for right now, it seems that we're on our own.

It goes without saying that it is imperative to install an effective water filter for your drinking water, a shower filter and, even better, a whole house water filter.

So, if we can't rely on the municipal water treatment systems, it's really up to each person to find solutions. It is obvious that homes, restaurants, hospitals, schools and businesses must realize the importance of providing not only pesticide and heavy metal free water, but also PPCP free water.

It has been shown that the most effective water purification system for removing all these contaminants, including PPCPs, is an activated carbon filtration system. There are units, which can filter your tap water, but it would be far wiser to install a whole home unit. Investing in this kind of system is your best protection for yourself and your family.

I personally use an excellent, affordable system called Aquasana. It has an exclusive dual filter system which uses a combination of carbon filtration, ion exchange and sub micron filtration to produce truly healthy water. It is capable of filtering out chlorine, lead, prescription drugs, pharmaceuticals, VOCs, MTBE and cysts (chlorine-resistant parasites) and, unlike other systems, leaves in the natural trace minerals!

Our bodies deserve only the purest water. Until the day comes when our water supply is again pristine, using a good filtration system has become one of the facts of 21st century life.

Chapter 14

The Total Body Detox Solution

The benefits of our modern way of life are many, but they come with a price—the pollution of our planet. The silent killers of the 21st century turn out to be the toxic heavy metals and chemicals that accumulate in our bodies over our lifetime.

The legacy of the past century was the creation of more than 80,000 chemicals. Each year the U.S releases a staggering 4 billion pounds of these toxins into our environment contaminating the air, water, soil, plants, animals, and of course, humans.

Mercury, lead, cadmium, arsenic, pesticides, insecticides, dioxins, furans, phthalates, VOCs and PCBs are just some for the foreign substances that have created an excessive body burden of harmful chemicals.

Just how bad is it? Pretty bad. Most of us have between 400-800 potentially toxic, carcinogenic, endocrine-disrupting and gene-damaging chemicals stored within our cells. Fetuses now grow in a womb contaminated with as many as 287 foreign chemicals. And more than 630,000 of the 4 million babies born in the United States are at risk for brain damage and learning difficulties due to mercury exposure in the womb. In fact, the level of mercury in umbilical-cord blood is 1.7 times higher than the level in the mother's blood!

Is the cancer epidemic related to toxins? According to the Columbia University School of Public Health, 95 percent of cancer is caused by poor diet and environmental toxicity.

And it's not just cancer. The systems most affected by these toxic compounds include the immune, neurological, and endocrine systems. Toxicity in these systems can lead to many chronic health problems including immune dysfunction, autoimmunity, asthma, allergies, autism, breast cancer, cognitive deficits, Chronic Fatigue Syndrome, early puberty, endometriosis, miscarriage, mood changes, neurological illnesses, obesity, lack of libido, hypothyroidism, reproductive dysfunction, and glucose dysregulation.

Of all the toxic exposures, mercury is without a doubt the most destructive. It is a deadly neurotoxin causing psychological, neurological, enzymatic and immunological problems. Mercury contributes to or causes all known illnesses including autism, autoimmune diseases, Alzheimer's disease, cancers, heart disease, endocrine problems, neurological and behavioral disorders.

The problem with toxins such as mercury and lead is that once they enter the body, they are difficult to remove. Toxic accumulation quickly overwhelms the body's detoxification pathways and can ultimately result in severe symptoms or a chronic, debilitating illness.

The alarming fact is that there are simply no safe levels of exposure to any of these toxic contaminants.

One More Piece to the Toxicity Puzzle

A respected pioneer in the field of heavy metal detoxification, Dr. Dietrich Klinghardt, M.D., PhD has determined that there is a direct correlation between stored toxins and infectious pathogens. He states that "for each equivalent of stored toxins there is an equal amount of pathogenic microorganisms in the body." The presence of stored toxins causes immune system deficiency that supports the growth of pathogens such as bacteria, viruses, fungi and parasites.

He has demonstrated that "pathogenic microorganisms tend to set up their housekeeping in the body compartments that have the highest pollution with toxic metals. The body's own immune cells are incapacitated in those areas whereas the microorganisms multiply and thrive in an undisturbed way."

For each equivalent of stored toxins there is an equal amount of pathogenic microorganisms in the body. Thus the importance of both treating infection and detoxifying simultaneously as part of a well-planned health optimization strategy cannot be understated.

The term Toxic Body Burden (TBB) is now being used in reference to synthetic toxic chemicals, heavy metals and pathogens that enter and accumulate in the body. Retaining and restoring health requires an effective two-pronged approach that can detoxify toxic substances while simultaneously eliminating infectious microorganisms.

Zeolite – Removes Toxins Naturally

Zeolite is a naturally occurring crystalline structure created from volcanic ash that spewed into the atmosphere during violent eruptions over 300 million years ago. For thousands of years, civilizations throughout the world have used zeolite as a traditional medicine.

What makes zeolite so unique is its cage-like, honeycombed structure, which is negatively charged. When ingested, this natural mineral attracts and irreversibly binds and removes toxic heavy metals, chemical elements and free radicals through the urinary tract. This process is called Chelation.

Many toxic poisons are positively charged and these toxins are attracted into the zeolite cage like the strong attraction of steel filings to a magnet.

One of the most significant benefits of zeolite over other detoxification agents is its affinity schedule for toxic heavy metals. Zeolite binds with mercury first and lead second, moving on to additional toxic heavy metals and chemical toxins which may include pesticides, herbicides, plastics and even radioactive particles, without removing precious nutrients such as calcium and magnesium.

However, zeolite goes far beyond the critical job of removing damaging toxins. Research has shown that it has many other vital actions in the body.

Zeolite removes free radicals. Unlike classic antioxidants, zeolite does not neutralize free radicals by donating an electron to stabilize them. Instead, zeolite's structure captures free radicals. Once trapped in the zeolite, the inactivated free radical can then safely be eliminated from the body.

Zeolite has broad-spectrum antiviral properties fighting viral infections in two ways: First, by attracting and binding viral sub-particles, thereby interfering with viral replication and eliminating them from the body. Secondly, by inhibiting viral proliferation.

Zeolite helps support proper pH by establishing optimum pH levels of the blood between 7.35 to 7.45, supporting an active immune system and healthy brain function.

Zeolite may help to eliminate carcinogenic toxins from the body, especially a category of carcinogens called nitrosamines. The most common sources for these nitrates include processed meats, cigarettes, and beer, which are linked to pancreatic, stomach, and colon cancers.

Zeolite treats diarrhea, promotes healthy digestion and encourages nutrient absorption. Zeolite's ability to capture ammonium ions during digestion promotes a healthier and less toxic digestive system.

There is growing evidence that suggests zeolite is an immune modulator and can increase specific groups of T cells.

A Silver Lining Against Pathogens

What did doctors prescribe before the advent of antibiotics to combat infections? The medical profession used colloidal silver. In 1914 the medical journal, *Lancet* reported phenomenal results from silver use stating it to be absolutely harmless, non-toxic to humans, and highly germicidal. In 1929 over 5 million prescriptions for colloidal silver were issued in the United States. In fact, colloidal silver has proven itself useful against all species of fungi, parasites, bacteria, protozoa, and viruses.

For centuries dating back to Hippocrates, silver's healing properties for both external and internal use for a variety of medical conditions was widely known. Properly formulated colloidal silver is beyond a shadow of a doubt, one of the most powerful, yet totally safe, antibiotics known to man.

With antibiotic resistant strains of bacteria increasing at an alarming rate, efficacious and advanced forms of colloidal silver are once again offering safe solutions.

The Total Body Detox Solution

To effectively address our Toxic Body Burden of harmful toxins and infections, SolutionsI.E. has created Total Body Detox comprising two revolutionary Intra-oral spray formulas called Total Zeolite and Total Silver.

Total Zeolite has many significant qualities which make it a superior choice over other detoxification or chelation methods, including other zeolite-based products. In urine challenge studies, Total Zeolite has been independently proven to increase urinary output of mercury, lead and other toxic metals by over 300 percent. It is interesting to note that extremely toxic mercury levels were recorded in the urine of patients while taking Total Zeolite who had undetectable mercury levels in their urine prior. These significant research results show just how difficult it is for the body to remove mercury and other toxins without an effective chelator present. Urine challenge (pre and post-provocation) studies are the gold standard in measuring the efficacy of any chelating agent.

Traditional chelating agents have significant limitations in safely removing mercury, lead, cadmium and arsenic. One drawback is that agents such as endrate (EDTA) have high affinity for essential nutrient minerals such as calcium and remove them simultaneously with toxins. If not carefully monitored, this removal of calcium can be quite dangerous and bring on rapid muscle weakness and potentially cause heart damage.

A distinct advantage of Total Zeolite is its highly selective attraction for toxic heavy metals with no attraction for vital nutrient minerals like calcium, potassium and selenium. However, its highest affinity is for mercury and lead.

Total Zeolite safely removes Mercury, Lead, Tin, Cadmium, Arsenic, Aluminum, Antimony, Nickel and all other toxic heavy metals.

With Total Zeolite toxins are tightly and irreversibly bound within the zeolite cage and safely eliminated though the urinary tract from the body within hours.

Another quality which makes ACZ nano® such an effective chelating agent is a proprietary nano-technology which provides significantly greater the number of nanomized zeolite crystals per dose. This results in an exponentially greater zeolite surface area providing far more attraction and elimination of toxins than other chelation products.

Total Zeolite is also the only zeolite product manufactured using wetter-water©, a proprietary aqueous solution that is 43 percent lower in surface tension than natural water. This allows micronutrients to be more effectively absorbed through the mucosa to rapidly enter into the blood plasma, continue through the interstitial spaces and into the cells.

Beyond the ability of Total Zeolite to remove toxins from the body, it boosts the immune system, enhances the body's metabolic function and nutrient absorption, alkalizes the body, and improves the body's ability to resist disease.

Total Zeolite is demonstrated to be so safe that it can even be used by pregnant mothers, children, or the elderly.

Total Silver — A Dynamic Duo

The partner in this dynamic duo is a unique silver-based antimicrobial Total Silver. Extremely effective, Total Silver demonstrates a much broader spectrum pathogen kill than traditional prescription antibiotics, antifungal, or antiviral preparations. Far more advanced in both safety and efficacy than traditional colloidal silver, Total Silver is a 200 PPM (parts per million) cellular silver, and has been proven capable of rapidly killing an enormous array of disease causing organisms—literally oxidizing the cell wall of gram positive and gram negative bacteria as well as naked virus, fungus and all without damaging human tissue. Independent studies show just how powerful Total Silver is, achieving complete kill against Methicillin-resistant Staphylococcus aureus (MRSA) and Candida in less than 3 minutes!

Cleanse and Live Vibrantly!

It is possible to live with severe Toxic Body Burden and still not "feel" toxic. This is the equivalent to driving down the freeway at 75 mph with bald tires. Everything seems fine until one of the tires blows. Countless victims of cancer and other life threatening diseases felt fine the day they were diagnosed. This is why toxins and pathogens are called invisible killers.

Cleansing your body now is crucial to maintaining health. The healing powers of nature enhanced with 21st century technology has created Total Zelote and Total Silver—the most effective, safe and affordable solution for the two greatest threats to optimal health today—chemical toxicity and chronic infections.

Chapter 15

The Wireless Dilemma: Hormone Disruption, Breast Cancer and Cell Phones

A defining moment in world history occurred in 1879 when Thomas Edison switched on the first light bulb. The flick of that switch radically transformed our world forever. The Age of Electricity was born.

Our love affair with all things electrical means that we are now living in a dense sea of electro-magnetic energy waves, called electro-magnetic radiation (EMR) which are estimated to be 100-200 million times greater than a hundred years ago!

Compounding the problem is the explosion of wireless technology such as cell phones, Bluetooth, PDA's, Wireless Internet, WiFi and powerful microwave emitting towers that are required for transmission. This pervasive wireless world emits a particular spectrum of electromagnetic radiation that has its own damaging effects on living systems.

Within just 2 decades, wireless technology has exploded onto the global scene. Presently, more than 236 million Americans, 20 million Canadians and 19 million Australians own a cell phone. More than 80 percent of the entire planet is connected to the wireless internet and by 2010, it will be 90 percent.

Our homeostasis is now being thrown into turmoil by unprecedented levels of all forms of EMR, seriously compromising our body's ability to properly function.

Anatomy of Electropollution 101

The 100 trillion cells of the human body communicate with each other by subtle low electromagnetic signals as well as through biochemical reactions. These signal pathways carry the information that becomes translated into all the biochemical and physiological processes of the body. Continuous exposure to electromagnetic radiation can drastically distort and disrupt these cellular communication pathways resulting in abnormal cellular metabolism and, ultimately, disease.

Electropollution-induced biological stress, profoundly compromises normal physiology and intercellular communication. Imagine the chaos that results when communication systems go down in a city. In the body, on a cellular level, a similar chaos is created when normal processes shut down and intercellular communication is disrupted. Cell function deteriorates; cell membranes harden; free radical damage occurs, nutrients can't get in and toxins can't get out. The break down of healthy cellular processes leads to biological chaos in our bodies.

Hundreds of studies have shown the harmful effects of EMR on the immune system, enzyme syntheses, nervous system , learning, moods and behavioral patterns. All aspects of life at the molecular, cellular, biochemical and physiological levels can potentially be damaged by EMR exposure.

Hormones, Cell Phones and Electropollution

Hormones are powerful substances. They pack a big wallop considering the tiny amounts that are produced by the endocrine glands. Most hormones such as estrogen, progesterone, testosterone, insulin and melatonin are made in parts per billion or parts per trillion. Even small hormonal fluctuations can create major physiological changes. As profound orchestrators of all of life's processes, maintaining hormonal balance is imperative for optimum health. When delicate hormonal balance and rhythms are altered, the body's ability to regulate fundamental systems goes haywire.

Our modern lifestyle poses many threats to optimal endocrine function. Stress, toxicity, poor quality food, lack of sleep, pharmaceutical medications are all known hormone disruptors. However, there is one particular kind of hormone disruptor that has been seriously overlooked—electromagnetic radiation.

Embedded deep within our brain is a light sensitive endocrine gland called the pineal gland, which is about the size of a pea. Since ancient times, the pineal gland was associated with the mystical all-seeing "Third Eye". Once dismissed as a useless gland, the pineal, which is, in fact, a light sensitive organ, is now considered to be one of the most significant glands in the body.

The pineal gland is the primary source of the hormone, melatonin. Discovered 50 years ago, it is now hailed as a miraculous hormone regulating many key functions of human growth and health and providing powerful anti-cancer protection. Melatonin is produced about 90 minutes after falling asleep. Studies have shown that blood concentrations of the hormone rise after dark from low daytime values and usually peak in the middle of the night.

Researchers are increasingly surprised at the extent of the physiological processes that are either controlled or influenced by melatonin: it regulates our circadian rhythms governing our waking/sleep cycle and it is one of the most efficient destroyers of free radicals thereby ensuring normal DNA synthesis and cell division to occur. Melatonin not only inhibits the release of estrogen but also actually suppresses the development of breast cancer. Melatonin's other anticancer property is its ability to increase the cytotoxicity of the immune system's killer lymphocytes. It is even is able to enhance the immune system and counteract stress-induced immunosuppression.

Melatonin's breast cancer fighting ability also addresses two other threats that can increase cell division in the breast— the hormone prolactin and the growth factor known as "epidermal growth factor".

Melatonin also enhances the tumor-fighting power of Vitamin D and increases this vitamin's ability to stop tumor growth. In fact, it makes Vitamin D's tumor fighting abilities 20-100 times stronger. In addition, melatonin acts as an aromatase inhibitor, a powerful protection against estrogen dependent cancers.

Needless to say, it is vital to ensure our body's ability to produce regular and adequate levels of melatonin on a daily basis. Unfortunately, sleeping in a room in which we are surrounded by all our favorite devices i.e. cordless or cell phones, digital clocks, CD/radio players, computers and TV's can seriously suppress our nightly melatonin production.

Japan's National Institute for Environmental Studies showed that breast cancer cells treated with melatonin would resume growing when exposed to power-frequency EMRs. It was found that magnetic fields disrupt the cells' signaling system, their internal communications network, which determines how they respond to their environment.

The EMR effect at 12mG was pretty much the same as the one from a field a hundred times higher at 1G. In fact, the effect was even stronger at the lower EMR dose than the higher one.

This mechanism has helped to explain why reduced melatonin levels from EMR has shown to cause a number of cancers including breast cancer, prostate cancer, colorectal cancer, melanoma, ovarian malignancies and childhood leukemia.

It is now known that melatonin suppression occurs at frequencies not far above those of the common household ranges of 50-60 hertz. If we sleep next to a cordless phone base station and/or digital clock or we have faulty electrical wiring, enough continuous EMR exposures are emitted to suppress nighttime melatonin production.

The connection between breast cancer and EMR continues to strengthen. Dr. Patricia Coogan at the Boston University of Public Health reported a 43 percent increased risk in women with a high likelihood of occupational exposure to magnetic fields such as those given off by mainframe computers. In fact, women who work in electrical jobs, including electricians, telephone installers, power line workers and electrical engineers have a greater risk of dying from breast cancer. This increased incidence has been directly linked to the suppression of melatonin from EMR

It's not just women that should be concerned about EMR's causal link to breast cancer. In five studies, elevated EMR have been implicated in an increased incidence of male breast cancer. Men who worked as telephone linemen, in switching stations, in the utilities industry were found to have as much as a sixfold increase in breast cancer.

More Hormone Disruption

Experimental physiologist, Dr. Charles Graham's research found that magnetic fields had an effect on two other hormones. Overnight exposure of women to elevated levels of EMR in the laboratory significantly increased estrogen levels, which is a known risk factor for breast cancer. In men, EMR exposure reduced levels of testosterone—a hormone drop that has been linked to testicular and prostate cancers.

Graham notes that a field's steady magnitude matters less than its intermittency or other features, such as power surges called electrical transients. These surges can pack a big burst of energy into a short period of time. They occur whenever lights or other electric devices turn on, when motors or compressors (such as those in refrigerators and air conditioners) cycle on, or when dimmer switches operate. Transients are hard to avoid because they may stem from surges elsewhere in a neighbor's house or even power lines up the street.

He also believes that EMR may actually fit the definition of an endocrine disrupter better than many hormone mimicking environmental pollutants because magnetic fields appear to elicit their effects by acting on and through hormones, rather than as hormones.

Millions of women around the world are prescribed tamoxifen, the most popular drug given to prevent recurrence of breast cancer. A very significant study showed that tamoxifen lost its ability to halt the proliferation of cancer cells when exposed to EMR. The level of EMR which produced this effect (12mG or more) is found in common sources such as a hair-dryer, vacuum cleaner, can openers, computers, microwave ovens, desk lamps, blenders and electric clocks.

Furthermore, while melatonin successfully reduced the growth rate of human breast cancer in culture, when exposed to 12mG, melatonin completely lost its ability to inhibit breast cancer cell growth.

Women, who are being treated for breast cancer with ta-moxifen are rarely, if ever, advised to reduce exposure to EMR or to use adequate technologies to protect themselves from EMR exposure.

Neurotransmitters, a special class of hormones which include serotonin and dopamine, play a major role in moods. Changes in serotonin levels are known to be associated with depression. For example, lowered levels of this chemical in the brain have been linked to an increase in suicide frequency. One study examined the brain functions of monkeys exposed to 60 Hz magnetic fields. It was found that the levels of serotonin and were significantly depressed immediately following ex-posure, and that only the dopamine returned to normal levels after several months.

Cortisol, Stress and What's in the Airways

Exposure to high levels of EMR also increases the levels of adrenaline, the flight or fight hormone, released from the adrenals glands B. Blake Levitt, author of *Electrical Fields*, states that, "Prolonged chronic stress is detrimental to every anatomical system, including the reproductive one. Subliminal stress may effect fertility and elevate blood pressure, which can lead to heart disease and strokes, as well as suppress im-mune function.... even short EMR exposures, like the use of a cordless phone on and off throughout the day, could cause spikes in such hormone levels."

The other stress hormone is cortisol, which affects long

term stress response. Also produced by the adrenals, cortisol is involved in glucose metabolism, regulating blood pressure, insulin release, inflammatory response and immune system function. Cortisol levels influence energy, memory, immune functions, and hormone balance. It should come as no surprise that EMR exposure has been found to cause increased serum cortisol.

Three Pieces of the Intervention Puzzle

Resolving the electropollution problem necessitates technologies that address three distinct interventions, i.e. primary, secondary and tertiary. All three levels of intervention are required in order to be adequately protected against electropollution.

Primary intervention technologies are those that act to prevent the cell membrane protective response from being inappropriately triggered. These act on the "cause" of the problems and include: headsets, active noise field technology (developed by the U.S. military) and passive noise field technologies.

Secondary intervention technologies are those that act to restore intercellular communication and thus can ameliorate the "effects" of the exposure to EMR. These are most effective in conjunction with primary interventions and include: subtle energy technologies, diodes and some pendants.

Tertiary intervention technologies are those that act to rehabilitate and correct cell damage. These work only in conjunction with primary and secondary intervention technologies and include: a nutrient rich diet and nutritional supplements such as antioxidants.

To ensure the greatest protection, all three "layers" must be initiated simultaneously: protect the cells from direct harm, re-establish healthy cell-to-cell communication and provide the body with the essential nourishment so it can repair itself and stay healthy.

It is imperative use technology that can address all three levels of intervention.

I have been seeking technology that can provide the best protection addressing all three interventions. The scientifically substantiated technology that I personally use is made by GIA Wellness. The patented and propriety technology called MRET (Molecular Resonant Technology) and ERT (Energy Resonsant Technology) offers proven protection against electropollution by protecting the cells from damage, improving cell-to-cell communication and repair cell damage.

As we rush head long into our exciting high tech world, we must also understand that we are all participating in a massive experiment. Electropollution is a very real threat to present and future generations. Effective interventions are not a luxury but simply a necessity. Like it or not the ever expanding and intrusive EMR world is here to stay. The responsibility lies with each one of us to take the proactive steps that will protect us, our family and future generations.

Chapter 16

Practical Protocols for Women's Health

Supporting our body with optimal nutrition is fundamental not only for our health but also essential for hormonal balance. The foods that most Americans consume on a daily basis would not fit my definition of nutritious fare.

If you truly want to regain hormonal balance, then the Hormone Wreckers must be radically reduced or, even better, eliminated from your diet and replaced by the health-promoting Hormone Harmonizers.

In this protocol section I will be suggesting nutritional supplements to support the most common hormone and health concerns of women. It is worth repeating that the basis for any healing program necessitates a healthy, nutrient-dense, organic (as much as possible) diet founded on the Hormone Harmonizers list.

Hormone Wreckers

1. Sugar and artificial sweeteners including all forms of cane sugar (even organic), pasteurized honey, Splenda, aspartame and agave syrup

2. Refined carbohydrates

3. Gluten grains: wheat, rye, barley, spelt, couscous, kamut

4. Sodas and all diet sodas, caffeine, alcohol

5. Toxic fats: all refined oils, margarine, canola oil, sunflower oil, safflower oil

6. Processed foods

7. Dehydration

8. Genetically Modified Organisms mostly found in soy, canola, papaya, corn

9. Electropollution from cell phones, wireless technologies and EMFs

Hormone Harmonizers

1. Healthy sweeteners: that do not spike blood sugar levels: stevia, xylitol, lo han, "Just Like Sugar", raw and unfiltered honey

2. Whole grains and seeds

3. Gluten-free grains and seeds: rice, millet, quinoa, buckwheat, Salba, hemp

4. Filtered water and naturally sweetened juices, natural sodas, healthy coffee substitutes (Teeccino), alcohol-free wines

5. Health fats: flax seed oil, Salba seed oil, hemp seed oil coconut oil olive oil, grapeseed oil, macadamia oil, butter, ghee

6. Organic foods (fruits, vegetables, oils, nuts, seeds, dairy and grassfed meats)

7. Seeds and Nuts: sesame seed, sunflower, pumpkin, almond, Brazil, walnut, pecan, hazelnut, cashew

8. Cultured and fermented foods: yogurt, kefir, sauerkraut, pickles, kim chee, miso

9. Celtic sea salt or Himalayan salt

10. Dark, unsweetened chocolate, cacao nibs

11. Filtered or spring water

12. GMO-foods — must be labeled GMO-free or organic

13. Electropollution Protection from cell phones, wireless technologies and EMFs (GIA Wellness products)

Recommended Nutritional Protocols

Health issues are always a communication from the body letting us know that something is out of balance. We may be too toxic, too physically or emotionally stressed, or too deficient in essential nutrients. Specific problems may require targeted nutrition or supplementation. The following protocols offer suggestions for an effective nutritional program to help address the most common women's health problems.

Breast Cancer Prevention

Multivitamin and Mineral Complex (Organic Life Vitamins by Natural Vitality)

Vitamin D3 – 2000-5000 IU daily

Proteolytic Enzymes – 600 mg, 3x daily between meals

Milk Thistle – 175 mg, 2 caps twice daily

Turmeric (Jarrow Curcumin 95) – 380 mg, 1-5x daily

Inositol – 100 mg

Chaste Tree Berry – 100 to 175 mg

Essential fatty acids from: fish oils, Salba seed oil or hemp seed oil (1000-3000 mg)

Green tea or green tea extract (3 cups of Herbabgreen Tea)

Lycopene – 10 mg

Iodoral (iodine) – 1 tablet twice daily

Sulfurophanes – (BroccoMax by Jarrow Formulas) 500 mg, 1-2 daily

Probiotics – Theralac – take twice a week (Master Supplements, Inc.) or Fem-Dophilus – take daily (Jarrow Formulas)

Candida Yeast Infections

Multivitamin and Mineral Complex (Organic Life Vitamins by Natural Vitality)

Vitamin K-2 – 60-80 mcg

Essential fatty acids from: fish oils, Salba seed oil or hemp seed oil (1000-3000 mg)

Naturcillin, a proprietary herbal blend, by Bio-Botanicals – start with 5 drops and go up to 5-7 drops three times a day or 10 twice a day.

Olive leaf Extract – Naturvirex by Bio-Botanicals one am and pm (works best in combination with Naturcillin)

Caprylic acid – 1-2 grams daily with meals

Oil of Oregano – 3 drops, 3x a day in juice or water

Probiotics – Theralac – take twice a week (Master Supplements, Inc.) or Fem-Dophilus – take daily (Jarrow Formulas)

Only use healthy sweeteners – xylitol, stevia, "Just Like Sugar"

Detoxification Support

Detox Clay Powder – topical and internal use (Living Clay)

Detox Cleansing Deodorant® – for daytime and nighttime use (Herbalix Restoratives)

MAX GXL Glutathione Accelerator (Thriving Health and Wellness)

Setria® Glutathione – Kyowa Hakko

Total Body Cleanse® – Total Silver and Total Zeolite (Solutions IE)

Endometriosis

Multivitamin and Mineral Complex (Organic Life Vitamins by Natural Vitality)

Natural progesterone cream 20 mg morning and night between days 7-26 if menstruating and 3 weeks on a week off if not menstruating (Only use paraban-free brands i.e. ProgestaPlus, EssProL'eve, ProGest or EndoPure)

Chromium picolinate – 200 mcg

Chaste Tree Berry – 100-175 mg

Proteolytic Enzymes – 600 mg, 3x daily between meals

Essential fatty acids from: fish oils, Salba seed oil or hemp seed oil (1000-3000 mg)

Curcumin Complex (Jiva Supplements) – 2 capsules, 3x daily

Evening Primrose oil – 3000 mg per day

Vitamin C with bioflavonoids – 2,000 mg, 3x daily

Beta Carotene – 5,000 units

Sulfurophanes – (BroccoMax by Jarrow Formulas) – 500 mg, 1-2 daily

Vitamin E – 400-2,000 IU daily as mixed tocopherols and tocotrienols or wheat germ oil

Iodoral (iodine) – 1 tablet twice daily

Probiotics – Theralac – take twice a week (Master Supplements, Inc.) or Fem-Dophilus – take daily (Jarrow Formulas)

Fibrocystic Breast Disease

Multivitamin and Mineral Complex (Organic Life Vitamins by Natural Vitality)

Iodoral (iodine) – 1 tablet twice daily

Essential fatty acids from: fish oils, Salba seed oil or hemp seed oil (1000-3000 mg)

Turmeric (Jarrow Curcumin 95) – 380 mg, 1-5x daily

Probiotics – Theralac – take twice a week (Master Supplements, Inc.) or Fem-Dophilus – take daily (Jarrow Formulas)

Fibroids

Please read the chapter on Healing Fibroids on page 215.

In addition I recommend using the following products by Jiva Supplements:

Curcumin & Fermented Soy Plus (Jiva Supplements)

Begin with 2 capsules 3x daily, after 3-5 days increase to 3 capsules 3x daily, and then increase again after 3-4 days to 4 capsules 3x daily until fibroids decrease

Fermented Soy and Curcumin Nutritional Beverage (Jiva Supplements) 1 scoop daily for small fibroids and 2 scoops for large fibroids.

Heart Disease Prevention

Multivitamin and Mineral Complex (Organic Life Vitamins by Natural Vitality)

Essential fatty acids from: fish oils, Salba seed oil or hemp seed oil (1000-3000 mg)

Probiotics – Theralac – take twice a week (Master Supplements, Inc.) or Fem-Dophilus – take daily (Jarrow Formulas)

Vitamin E – 400-2,000 IU daily as mixed tocopherols and tocotrienols or wheat germ oil

Magnesium (Natural Calm by Natural Vitality) – 400-800 mg

Potassium citrate – 500 mg per day

Coenzyme Q10 (QH-Absrob by Jarrow Formulas) – 1 to 3 softgels daily with meals

Proteolytic Enzymes – 600 mg, 3x daily between meals

Pomegranate Antioxidants (CardioPom by Pomegranate Health) – 2 capsules daily

Hawthorn extract – 100-200 mg, 3x daily

Garlic – 2000-4000 mg

Gugulipid – 500 mg, 3x daily

Vitamin D3 – 2000-5000 IU daily

Adrenal Support – Dr. Wilson's Dynamite Adrenals by Nutricology, 2-4 scoops daily

Osteoporosis

Multivitamin and Mineral Complex (Organic Life Vitamins by Natural Vitality)

Essential fatty acids from: fish oils, Salba seed oil or hemp seed oil (1000-3000 mg)

Probiotics – Theralac – take twice a week (Master Supplements, Inc.) or Fem-Dophilus – take daily (Jarrow Formulas)

Silicon – 6-10 drops dail (JarroSil by Jarrow Formulas)

Complete bone nutrient support (Bone-Up by Jarrow Formulas) 2-3x daily or OsteoCalm (Natural Vitality) – 1/2 cap twice a day

Natural progesterone cream 20 mg morning and night between days 7-26 if menstruating and 3 weeks on a week off if not menstruating (Only use paraban-free brands i.e. ProgestaPlus, EssProL'eve, ProGest or EndoPure)

Theanine – Relaxing Tea (Herbasway) or Zen Mind (Nutricology)

Adrenal Support – Dr. Wilson's Dynamite Adrenals by Nutricology, 2-4 scoops daily

Ovarian Cysts

Multivitamin and Mineral Complex (Organic Life Vitamins by Natural Vitality)

Milk Thistle – 175 mg, 2 caps twice daily.

Calcium D-glucarate – 150-300 mg

Turmeric (95% curcumin) – 5-100 mg

Chaste Tree Berry – 100-175 mg

Evening Primrose oil – 3000 mg per day

Green tea extract – 100-200 mg

Iodoral (iodine) – 1 tablet twice daily

Proteolytic Enzymes – 600 mg, 3x daily between meals

Sulforaphane (found in cruciferous vegetables) – 100 mcg-200 mcg

Natural progesterone cream – use 20 mg morning and night between days 14-26 if menstruating and 3 weeks on a week off if not menstruating (Only use paraban-free brands i.e. ProgestaPlus, EssProL'eve, ProGest or EndoPure)

Theanine – Relaxing Tea (Herbasway) or Zen Mind (Nutricology)

Perimenopause and Menopause Support

(Estrogen dominance, hot flashes, mood swings, fatigue, headaches, insomnia, etc.)

Multivitamin and Mineral Complex (Organic Life Vitamins by Natural Vitality)

Vitamin A – 2,500 IU Daily

Vitamin C – 2000 mg, 4x daily

Vitamin E – 400-2,000 IU daily as mixed tocopherols and tocotrienols or wheat germ oil

Vitamin C with bioflavonoids – 2,000 mg, 3x daily

Black cohosh – 80-160 mg of standardized extract a day

Milk Thistle – 175 mg, 2 caps 2x daily

Digestive Enzymes (Jarro-Zymes) – 1 with each meal

Maca (Maca Plus by International Health) – 900 mg

Natural progesterone cream 20 mg morning and night between days 7-26 if menstruating and 3 weeks on a week off if not menstruating (Only use paraban-free brands i.e. ProgestaPlus, EssProL'eve, ProGest or EndoPure)

Adrenal Support – Dr. Wilson's Dynamite Adrenals by Nutricology, 2-4 scoops daily

Pomegranate Extract – 400 mg, 2-3x daily (Pomegranate Health)

Sulfurophanes – (BroccoMax by Jarrow Formulas) 500 mg, 1-2x daily

High Potency B complex – 50-100 mg

Essential fatty acids from: fish oils, Salba seed oil or hemp seed oil (1000-3000 mg)

Theanine – Relaxing Tea (Herbasway) or Zen Mind (Nutricology)

Polycystic Ovarian Syndrome (PCOS)

Multivitamin and Mineral Complex (Organic Life Vitamins by Natural Vitality)

Essential fatty acids from: fish oils, Salba seed oil or hemp seed oil (1000-3000 mg)

Iodoral (iodine) – 1 tablet twice daily

Maca (Maca Plus by International Health) – 900 mg

Turmeric (Jarrow Curcumin 95) – 380 mg, 1-5x daily

Natural progesterone cream 20 mg morning and night between days 7-26 if menstruating and 3 weeks on a week off if not menstruating (Only use paraban-free brands i.e. ProgestaPlus, EssProL'eve, ProGest or EndoPure)

Probiotics – Theralac – take twice a week (Master Supplements, Inc.) or Fem-Dophilus – take daily (Jarrow Formulas)

Proteolytic Enzymes – 600 mg, 3x daily between meals

Premenstrual Syndrome

Multivitamin and Mineral Complex (Organic Life Vitamins by Natural Vitality)

Magnesium (Natural Calm by Natural Vitality) – 400-800 mg

B-Complex – 50-100 mg

Vitamin E – 400-2,000 IU daily as mixed tocopherols and tocotrienols or use pure wheat germ oil

Essential fatty acids from: fish oils, Salba seed oil or flaxseed oil – (1000-3000 mg)

Turmeric (Jarrow Curcumin 95) – 380 mg, 1-5x daily

Maca (Maca Plus by International Health) – 900 mg

Chaste Tree Berry – 100-175 mg

Evening Primrose oil – 3000 mg

Green tea extract – 100-200 mg or HerbaGreen Tea Concentrate, 1-3 droppersful daily

Sulfurophanes (BroccoMax by Jarrow Formulas) – 500 mg, 1-2x daily

Natural progesterone cream 20 mg morning and night between days 7-26 if menstruating and 3 weeks on a week off if not menstruating (Only use paraban-free brands i.e. ProgestaPlus, EssProL'eve, ProGest or EndoPure)

Vitamin C – 1000 mg, 2x daily

Probiotics – Theralac – take twice a week (Master Supplements, Inc.) or Fem-Dophilus – take daily (Jarrow Formulas)

Theanine – Relaxing Tea (Herbasway) or Zen Mind (Nutricology)

Adrenal Support – Dr. Wilson's Dynamite Adrenals by Nutricology, 2-4 scoops daily

Skin Problems

Multivitamin and Mineral Complex (Organic Life Vitamins by Natural Vitality)

Zinc – 5 mg

Selenium – 200 mcg

Vitamin A – 500 IU

Evening Primrose or Borage oil – 1000 mg

Essential fatty acids from: fish oils, Salba seed oil or hemp seed oil (1000-3000 mg)

Probiotics – Theralac – take twice a week (Master Supplements, Inc.) or Fem-Dophilus – take daily (Jarrow Formulas)

Garlic Allicin – 1000 mg

Chaste Tree Berry – 100-175 mg

Spotless Cream (USA Sprunk-Jansen)

Critical Care Holistic Healing Mist (Sunshine Botanicals)

Rescue Rapid Repair Serum (Sunshine Botanicals)

Stress, Anxiety Attacks and Night Sweats

Adrenal Support – Dr. Wilson's Dynamite Adrenals by Nutricology, 2-4 scoops daily

Magnesium (Natural Calm by Natural Vitality) – 400-1200 mg

Essential fatty acids from: fish oils, Salba seed oil or hemp seed oil (1000-3000 mg)

Turmeric (Jarrow Curcumin 95) – 380 mg, 1-5x daily

Probiotics – Theralac – take twice a week (Master Supplements, Inc.) or Fem-Dophilus – take daily (Jarrow Formulas)

Natural progesterone cream 20 mg morning and night between days 7-26 if menstruating and 3 weeks on a week off if not menstruating (Only use paraban-free brands i.e. ProgestaPlus, EssProL'eve, ProGest or EndoPure)

Vaginal Dryness and Atrophy

Multivitamin and Mineral Complex (Organic Life Vitamins by Natural Vitality)

Essential fatty acids from: fish oils, Salba seed oil or hemp seed oil (1000-3000 mg)

Vitamin E – 400-2,000 IU daily as mixed tocopherols and tocotrienols or wheat germ oil

Probiotics – Theralac – take twice a week (Master Supplements, Inc.) or Fem-Dophilus – take daily (Jarrow Formulas)

Pomegranate Seed Extract (MoisturePom by Pomegranate Health) – apply am and pm

Estriol Vaginal Cream (do not use if at risk of breast cancer) available from International Health

Chapter 17

Resources for Hormonal Balance and Optimal Health

This resource section lists the products that I use both for myself and in my clinical practice. While there are many excellent products available, I have chosen to include the specific ones that I know are the purest and most effective. My intention is to offer you a trustworthy source that can assist you in creating optimal health and wellness.

ANTIOXIDANT AND IMMUNE SUPPORT

CardioPom – 100% Pomegranate Antioxidant Formula

CardioPom is an all-natural blend of pure pomegranate fractions formulated to deliver the full spectrum of pomegranate's polyphenol antioxidants, such as punicalagins, ellagitannins, and flavonoids. These powerful antioxidants work synergistically to help reduce free radicals, maintain healthy cholesterol and blood pressure levels, and promote cardiovascular health. CardioPom delivers the antioxidant benefits of fresh pomegranate juice without the sugar.

Pomegranate Health
800-661-5176   www.pomhealth.com

CocoPure Chocolate Tea

In this delicious powdered drink you're getting 4000 mg of pure concentrated cocoa with elevated levels of flavonoids that offer a powerhouse of antioxidant protection against free radical damage. In addition, it is fortified with the cardio-supporting ingredients of Resveratrol, and all the protective qualities of Green Tea. It is sweetened with xylitol and stevia.

New Vitality
800-290-0221   www.NewVitality.com

Curcumin & Fermented Soy Plus

It is a patent pending proprietary formulation using patented curcumin, bioperine and organically grown, non-GMO fermented whole soy beans. It contains powerful anti-inflammatory properties to help support and maintain optimal bone, joint and cartilage health and other chronic inflammatory and degenerative conditions.

Jiva Supplements
800-517-7606   www.jivasupplements.org

Fermented Soy and Curcumin Nutritional Beverage

It is a patent pending proprietary researched formulation which contains the highest quality, non-GMO fermented whole soy protein, curcumin C3 complex and Bioperine. This unique phytonutrient formulation has powerful antioxidant properties and includes specific standardized ingredients that interact synergistically in maintaining optimal health for both men and women.

Jiva Supplements
800-517-7606   www.jivasupplements.org

HerbaGreen Tea

HerbaGreen Tea contains 90% polyphenols, 50% of which are EGCG (epigallocatechin gallate). Lotus leaf is rich in isoflavones. Kudzu helps to open the blood vessels. Lo Han and Stevia provide a balancing and moistening effect on internal organs. It effectively cleanses, nourishes, energizes and balances your body, giving you more vitality and better health. It comes in a variety of flavors.

Herbasway
800-672-7322   www.herbasway.com

Naturcillin

A laboratory tested, broad-spectrum botanical compound designed to support the entire immune system. Carefully crafted formula targets the intestines and supports digestion as well as immune function. Independent laboratory testing has concluded that it has broad reaching effects in challenging environments.

Bio-Botanicals Research Inc.

888-344-2144   www.naturcillin.com

Naturvirex

A proven botanical compound formulated around the successful attributes of Olive Leaf extract, this formula is specifically designed to support the immune systems activity while assisting in the removal of waste through the enhancement and promotion of detoxification. It is particularly useful in the treatment of virus, retrovirus, and bacterium or protozoa infection.

Bio-Botanicals Research Inc.

888-344-2144   www.naturcillin.com

NutraRev

It is a premium combination of popular anti-aging supplements to help offset the effects of aging, assist energy production, reduce fatigue and support heart health. It includes POMELLA® pomegranate, SolQ10BLUE™ CoQ-10 and Bioenergy RIBOSE™ along with acetyl-L-carnitine, alpha lipoic acid and vitamins C, E and B_6 and the antioxidants açaí, goji, mangosteen, grape, wild blueberry, raspberry, cranberry, prune, tart cherry, wild bilberry and strawberry.

Natural Vitality

800-446-7462   www.petergillham.com

PeakImmune4 Immune Complex

This is a dietary supplement, which contains 250 mg of Rice Bran Arabinoxylan Compound (RBAC), which has been scientifically shown to support the immune system. It is clinically shown to triple Natural Killer Cell Activity.

Daiwa Health Development, Inc.

866-475-4810   www.dhdusa.net

Pomegranate Tea Concentrate

It s a liquid concentrate formula, rich in anti-oxidants, derived from a proprietary mixture of pomegranate extracts and green tea extract. Using extracts of the whole fruit as well as the juice, Pomegranate offers you more than regular juice without sugar, artificial sweeteners or calories.

Herbasway
800-672-7322   www.herbasway.com

QH-Absorb

Ubiquinol is the reduced (active antioxidant) form of Co-Q10, the form that is directly used in human metabolism as a lipid-soluble antioxidant. The Ubiquinol of QSURGE™ formula directly provides the activated form, and also has superior bioavailability to ubiquinone, as demonstrated in clinical trials. It is a natural proliposome lipid-soluble delivery system, which has been clinically shown in humans to increase Co-Q10 levels up to 400 percent.

Jarrow Formulas
www.jarrow.com

BONE HEALTH

Bone-Up

It is a complete multinutrient bone-health system. It combines Microcrystalline Hydroxyapatite (MCHA) (from free-range Australian calves) with vitamin K2 as MK-7 (a more bioavailable form of vitamin K) and vitamin D3 to support the deposition of calcium into the bones as well as to assist in building up the organic bone matrix.* Potassium citrate is also added for optimal osteo support.

Jarrow Formulas
www.jarrow.com

JarroSil

This is a synergistic formulation of highly bioavailable silicon. Silicon plays an important role in bone calcification, including during the growth of new bone. It is an essential partner of calcium for bones, glucosamine for joints and antioxidants for supple and healthy arteries. It also improves the strength and elasticity of collagen by stimulating collagen production. Stronger collagen means healthier, more elastic skin, and fewer and shallower wrinkles.

Jarrow Formulas
www.jarrow.com

Osteo Calm

A premium bone health support supplement. It balances calcium with Magnesium in a natural orange-vanilla liquid with certified organic stevia and organic agave nectar. It features brand-name ingredients GloCal® calcium and Natural Calm® magnesium. Osteo Calm also includes vitamins to assist calcium absorption and support bone health (A, D3, B6, C, K2 and folic acid) and minerals in ionic form (zinc, copper, manganese, potassium and boron).

Natural Vitality
800-446-7462   www.petergillham.com

DETOXIFICATION SUPPORT

Detox Clay Powder

Detox your body safely with 9.7pH Living Clay®, a unique and rare, green swelling calcium Bentonite clay with Montmorillonite properties from the Smectite family of clays. Its astoundingly strong drawing action cleanses by pulling out impurities while its dynamic binding power captures and eliminates toxins. In addition, the clay's vibrant electromagnetic charge stimulates cellular revitalization. Also available as Cleansing Clay Mask, Body Cream, Wrinkle Release Cream and Bar Soaps.

Living Clay
800-915-2529   www.livingclayco.com

Detox Cleansing Deodorant®

This is the first nighttime Detox Cleansing Deodorant formulated and clinically tested to release trapped impurities from under the arm while you sleep. Companion daytime non-suppressive deodorants work to control perspiration and body odors for natural healthy hygiene. All products are free of synthetic chemicals and petroleum.

Herbalix Restoratives
866-387-4222   www.herbalixrestoratives.com

Total Body Cleanse® by SOLUTIONS IE®

Premature aging and nearly every chronic disease process is related to toxicity. Maintaining vibrant health requires an effective approach that can remove toxic substances and infectious microorganisms from the body.

Total Silver® is anti-fungal, anti-viral and bactericidal.
Total Zeolite binds and expels toxic heavy metals, free radicals and more.

Solutions IE
888-234-6863   www.solutionsie.com

GLUTATHIONE PRODUCTS

MaxGXL (Glutathione Accelerator)

MaxGXL provides the proper nutrients needed to promote the body's own ability to manufacture and absorb glutathione. **MaxGXL** also aids in liver support, thus helping the liver to function as the main production site and storehouse for glutathione.

Thriving Health and Wellness
415-885-7188   www.ThrivingHealthandWellness.com

Setria

Setria® Glutathione is a tripeptide consisting of three amino acids: glutamate, cysteine, and glycine. It is found to varying degrees in all cells, tissues, body fluids, and organ system. Dietary supplements of Setria glutathione can raise glutathione levels in critical tissues such as the lungs, intestines and kidneys, as well as blood plasma.

Kyowa Hakko http://setriaglutathione.com

GUT AND DIGESTIVE HEALTH

Enzalase
Contains 12 digestive enzymes in a high potency, acid-proof, deep release formulation, compatible with probiotics and helps support optimal digestion of fats, proteins and carbohydrates.

Master Supplements, Inc.
800-926-2961   www.theralac.com

Fem Dophilus
It is an oral probiotic for natural vaginal health. It contains two patented and clinically documented probiotic strains, *Lactobacillus rhamnosus* GR-1® and *Lactobacillus reuteri* RC-14® which helps to maintain or restore healthy vaginal flora that are important in maintaining vaginal health and support the health of the urinary tract.

Jarrow Formulas
www.jarrow.com

Theralac
It is a new, highly effective probiotic that replenishes beneficial bacteria that colonize the human intestinal tract with 40 billion CFU of five new generation probiotic strains. It also promotes a healthy soft lining (wall) in the intestinal tract, which results in improved digestion, regularity and nutrient absorption.

Master Supplements, Inc.
800-926-2961   www.theralac.com

TruFiber
It is a soluble fiber with Bifidogenic enzymes uniquely formulated to stimulate probiotics.

Master Supplements, Inc.
800-926-2961   www.theralac.com

HEALTHY HOME SOLUTIONS

Aquasana

Aquasana's dual filter system uses a combination of carbon filtration, ion exchange and sub micron filtration to produce healthy water from your kitchen tap. Filters out chlorine, lead, prescription drugs, pharmaceuticals, VOCs, MTBE and cysts (chlorine-resistant parasites) and leaves in the natural trace minerals.

Shower
The Shower Filter has a unique two-stage filter process. Stage 1 removes chlorine and enhances pH balance with a copper/zinc mineral media, and stage 2 uses a carbonized coconut shell for the removal of synthetic chemicals, THMs and VOCs that are inhaled or absorbed through the skin.

Whole House
The Rhino® EQ-300 Home Water Filtration System has 3 stages of filtration, effectively filtering out chlorine, sediment and synthetic chemicals for healthy water throughout your entire home!

If you mention either *Hormone Heresy* you will receive a 20% discount off all Aquasana systems.

Sun Water Systems, Inc.
866-662-6885   www.aquasana.com

ElectroPollution Protection
GIA Wellness offers a suite of products based on scientifically proven technologies to protect against the many harmful effects of electropollution from cell phones, cordless phones, wireless routers, computers and other wireless technologies.

WomanWise International
918-728-7069   www.whatwomenmustknow.com

HEALTHY SKIN

AgelessPom – A Pomegranate Seed Oil Blend

A premium food-grade pomegranate seed oil blend rich in powerful omega-5 conjugated fatty acids, omega-9 fatty acids, antioxidants, and gentle phytoestrogens that work together in a synergistic way to help revitalize the skin, resolves fine wrinkles, soothes minor skin irritations, and assists in restoring youthfulness.

Pomegranate Health
800-661-5176   www.pomhealth.com

Red Dry Skin

A natural topical skin care remedy to relieve the discomfort and distress of red, itchy, scaly skin such as found in eczema and psoriasis.

USA Sprunk-Jansen LLC
888-977-7865   www.sprunk-jansen.com

Spotless

A topical cream clears up blemishes and acne gently. This unique herbal formula eases redness reduces acne bacteria and oil production without drying or irritating.

USA Sprunk-Jansen LLC
888-977-7865   www.sprunk-jansen.com

Sunshine Botanicals

This award-winning range of products provides natural clinical skin care from a botanical perspective. It is totally free of parabens, gluten, phthalates, parabens, propylene glycol, ureas, EDTA, fragrances, petroleum, encapsulated nano particles, and artificial colors. Based on pure botanical ingredients, the complete range is able to regenerate mature skin, heal irritated, blemished skin and repair skin damaged by free radicals and environmental pollution.

866-907-9546   www.sunshinebotanicals.com

HEALTHY WEIGHT MANAGEMENT
The Ultimate Fat Loss and Body Rejuvenation Program with Homeopathic HCG

A comprehensive, safe program using homeopathic formulas to support the release of stored fat reserves and resculpting of the body. It is able to reset the hypothalamus, which helps to maintain long term weight loss.

WomanWise International
918-728-7069   www.whatwomenmustknow.com

Cholesterol Level

A scientifically proven herbal formula, which contains tow herb extracts, Japanese Loquat and Southern European Olive that have been clinically proven when combined will help support cholesterol levels.

USA Sprunk-Jansen LLC
888-977-7865   www.sprunk-jansen.com

Glucose Level

A scientifically-proven herbal formula which helps to support glucose metabolism and to maintain insulin levels. It uses four plant extracts — Nettle, Salt Bush, Walnut and Olive — which work together to help bring your blood sugar levels into alignment.

USA Sprunk-Jansen LLC
888-977-7865   www.sprunk-jansen.com

Weighlevel

A scientifically proven herbal formula, which contains four herb extracts that suppress your appetite and stimulate your metabolism, thus allowing your body to deal with food more effectively.

USA Sprunk-Jansen LLC
888-977-7865   www.sprunk-jansen.com

HORMONAL BALANCE

The following natural hormone support products are free of toxic preservatives such as parabens and other chemicals.

BalancePom

100% Pomegranate Hormone Balancing Formula
BalancePom contains a completely natural range of pure pomegranate fractions including antioxidant and estrogenic compounds that work synergistically to help promote and maintain healthy hormone balance.

Pomegranate Health
800-661-5176   www.pomhealth.com

BalancePom Plus (Pomegranate with Traditional Herbs) BalancePom Plus is the perfect combination of a completely natural range of pure pomegranate fractions—including antioxidant and estrogenic compounds that work synergistically to help promote and maintain healthy hormone balance with a well-balanced selection of traditional herbs known for their positive impact on women's health. BalancePom Plus can help boost libido and reduce the unwanted discomforts of hormonal imbalance, such as hot flashes, night sweats, and moodiness.

Pomegranate Health
800-661-5176   www.pomhealth.com

EndoPure Homeopathic Hormone Rejuvenation Products

They are a range of FDA registered homeopathic Hormone Rejuvenation products which includes EndoPure Pro (Progesterone Homeopathic), EndoPure Estro (Estrogen Homeopathic), EndoPure Testos-Female (Testosterone Homeopathic).

The Wellness Center
800-219-1261   www.wellnesscenter.net

EssProl'eve

EssProl'eve is a natural (plant-derived) progesterone cream free of fillers, artificial colors and chemicals.

International Health
800-481-9987   www.ihsite.com

Maca Plus

Maca supports hormonal balance and both male and female reproductive health. and also provides energy. Consists of 10 to 1 Pure Maca Root Extract, which naturally has high amounts of essential amino acids, fatty acids, vitamins and minerals.

International Health
800-481-9987   www.ihsite.com

Menstrual Comfort Cream

Menstrual Comfort Cream is an Over-the-Counter (OTC) topical, transdermal cream that provides immediate relief for menstrual cramps and aches.

Emerita Products
800-888-6041   www.emerita.com

Pro-Gest

Pro-Gest is a natural progesterone cream that assists women with the relief of issues related to perimenopause and menopause.

Emerita Products
800-888-6041   www.emerita.com

Phytoestrogen Body Cream

Phytoestrogen Body Cream contains phytoestrogens, plant-derived compounds that can produce mild estrogen-like effects, which helps women, balance their estrogen levels appropriately.

Emerita Products
800-888-6041   www.emerita.com

(P)ro-Gest (M)enstrual (S)olutions

(P)ro-Gest (M)enstrual (S)olutions is a bioidentical natural progesterone cream that assists women with the relief of issues related to Premenstrual Syndrome.

Emerita Products
800-888-6041   www.emerita.com

ProgestaPlus

ProgestaPlus has a unique formulation containing only natural organic ingredients including beneficial Liposomes* — not cosmetic oil carriers—to improve transdermal skin absorption. It has high quality natural, bio-identical progesterone with natural herbal ingredients.

Aarisse Health Care Products
800-675-9329   www.healthyhormones.com

Prosta-Health for Men

Men need progesterone, too! A Natural Progesterone Body Cream that includes herbs and vitamins to support prostate health, improved libido, and energy.

Aarisse Health Care Products
800-675-9329   www.healthyhormones.com

HORMONE TESTING
SALIVA TESTING AND BLOOD SPOT TESTING

ZRT Laboratory

ZRT Laboratory's state-of-the-art saliva and blood spot testing technology allows for accurate measurement of a broad array of hormones and detection of existing hormone imbalance.

Saliva Testing Convenient home collection, accurate, and inexpensive, Saliva Testing provides a true picture of the bio-available levels of steroid hormones. The following hormones can be tested: estradiol, progesterone. testosterone, DHEA and cortisol.

Blood Spot Testing offers an easy alternative to blood draws in the doctor's office. The process requires only blood from a nearly painless finger prick and several tests can be run from a single sample Tests offered in the Blood Spot Profiles include: steroid hormones, thyroid hormones, Prostate Specific

Antigen, Vitamin D 3, Hemoglobin A1c, High Sensitivity C-Reactive Protein insulin and cholesterols.

ZRT Laboratory
866-600-1636   www.zrtlab.com

INCREASED LIBIDO

Feminine

This formula is based on the ancient wisdom of the Greek-Arabic tradition of herbal remedies. There's evidence that the ancient Egyptians used the herb Asafoetida over 4,000 years ago. And it's been widely used in the Greek-Arabic herbal traditions for tiredness and to increase sexual desire. It also contains Capers, which have been traditionally used as an aphrodisiac.

USA Sprunk-Jansen LLC
888-977-7865   www.sprunk-jansen.com

NATURAL HEALTHY SWEETENERS

Just Like Sugar

It is a 100% natural FDA GRAS (generally recognized as safe) approved sweetener made from only the purest of ingredients. It comprises a perfect blend of Chicory Root Dietary Fiber, Vitamin C, Calcium and orange peel. It leaves no after taste, does not raise blood sugar and is great for all your baking and cooking needs. Best of all it tastes just like sugar.

Just Like Sugar, Inc.
866-547-8427   www.justlikesugarinc.com

NuStevia White Stevia

White Stevia Powder contains 60% more Stevia extract than most other brands and has no bitter aftertaste.

NuNaturals
800-753-4372   www.morefiber.net/sellman

NuStevia NoCarbs Blend

It uses Erythritol, a natural filler that is produced from corn. Erythritol enhances the taste of Stevia. NuStevia White Stevia NoCarbs will have absolutely no effect on blood sugar levels and is safe for both Type I and II diabetics.

MoreFiber Stevia Baking Blend Powder

As a dietary supplement use it in your favorite recipe. More-Fiber contains NuStevia, Maltodextrin, Dextrin Fiber, Oat Fiber, Acacia Gum, Tapioca Flour, Guar Gum & Xanthan Gum.

Sweet Xylitol Crystals

It is a naturally occurring 5-carbon polyol sweetener found in many fruits and vegetables. Xylitol is even produced by the human body during normal metabolism of glucose. Xylitol is the sweetest of all the polyols. It is as sweet as sucrose, has no after-taste and is safe for diabetics.

SPECIAL OFFER - If you mention Hormone Heresy, you will receive a 20% discount on all the products you purchase.

NuNaturals
800-753-4372   www.morefiber.net/sellman

NUTRITIONAL SUPPORT

Organic Life Vitamins

A blend of the finest ingredients including 24 whole food antioxidant vegetables, superfruits, berries and fruits including acai, mangosteen, goji berry, organic pomegranate and organic noni plus organic ACTIValoe™whole-leaf aloe vera, multiple vitamins, ConcenTrace® trace mineral complex, Natural Vitality Amino Acid Complex, OptiMSM® and Chromax® chromium picolinate. It is sweetened with organic agave nectar and organic stevia (no added fructose), has a great light berry taste (organic raspberry and cranberry.

Natural Vitality
800-446-7462   www.petergillham.com

Salba – Whole Seed Nature's richest whole food source of Omega-3's and Fiber. Sprinkle it on cereal and salads or mix it into sauces and soup.

Salba Seed Oil
Each 1 Tbsp serving contains over 8,300 mg of Omega-3s in an ideal 3-to-1 ratio, making it nature's richest whole food source of Omega-3s.

Salba Whole Food Bars (Cranberry Nut, Tropical Fruit, Mixed Berry) A great wholesome treat or energy bar with all-natural, premium whole food ingredients including a full 12 gram serving of Salba—nature's richest plant-based source of Omega-3s and Fiber.

Core Naturals
888-895-3603   www.salba.com

STRESS SUPPORT

Dr. Wilson's Dynamite Adrenals
Based on the work of Dr. James Wilson, this formula combines the important nutrients for optimal adrenal function and regeneration: adrenal and other glandulars, herbs, amino acids, vitamins and minerals.

NutriCology, Inc.
800-545-9960   www.nutricology.com

L-Theanine Relaxation Tea
L-Theanine Relaxation Tea is a balanced formula with standardized extracts of wild crafted herbs from the mountains of China and the fields of Europe. These herbs have been carefully selected and processed, according to HerbaSway's rigorous criteria, to provide you with the most potent therapeutic benefits. L-Theanine Relaxation Tea combines Chamomile extract, Passionflower extract, Magnesium and L-Theanine into a delicious, relaxing tea.

Herbasway
800-672-7322   www.herbasway.com

Natural Calm

The Anti-Stress Drink for restoring a healthy magnesium level and balancing calcium intake—the result of which is *natural stress relief*. It features a proprietary formula of highly absorbable, water-soluble magnesium citrate in ionic form. *Natural Calm* is available in original and flavored versions, which contain organic raspberry, lemon and/or orange flavors and organic stevia (no added fructose).

Natural Vitality
800-446-7462   www.petergillham.com

Thre' Energy

Thre' (pronounced "three") is a unique combination of energy producing herbs provide a healthy, all-natural alternative to the high sugar, high caffeine energy drinks on the market. Its ingredients include Bitter Orange for energy and stimulates fat burning, Eleuthero for mental acuity and physical vitality, the amino acid taurine for energy and Vitamin B12 to assist in the process of converting food energy.

Herbasway
800-672-7322   www.herbasway.com

ZenMind

ZenMind offers a unique and natural way to promote relaxation without sedation. This formula contains a combination of L-theanine and GABA. L-theanine, stimulates the production of alpha-wave activity in the brain and GABA is a neurotransmitter that enhances relaxation.

NutriCology, Inc.
800-545-9960   www.nutricology.com

VAGINAL DRYNESS

MoisturePom – Vaginal Ointment

MoisturePom provides an all-natural solution for women who suffer from vaginal dryness and its accompanying itching, burning and irritation. The ingredients in MoisturePom consist of pure, plant-derived oils, each of which naturally contains an array of nutrients that are easily absorbed, providing fatty acids and antioxidants directly to the vaginal tissue cells. MoisturePom was specifically created as an ointment, designed to provide maximum absorbability. Its formula is comprised of pure pomegranate oil—plus oils of cocoa butter, coconut and extra virgin olive. It uses no artificial lubricants or petrochemical coatings. MoisturePom has the ability to repair vaginal tissue, create increased natural moisture, and promote the integrity of the cells, as well as to help reverse the atrophy of vaginal tissue. It has similar benefits as estrogen but without any of the associated risks and side effects.

Pomegranate Health
800-661-5176   www.pomhealth.com

Chapter 18

Educational and Support Resources

Breast Cancer Fund
In response to the public health crisis of breast cancer, the Breast Cancer Fund identifies—and advocates for elimination of—the environmental and other preventable causes of the disease. Through public education, policy initiatives, outdoor challenges and other innovative campaigns, the Breast Cancer Fund mobilizes the public to secure the changes needed to stop this disease before it starts.

www.breastcancerfund.org

Environmental Health Perspectives
The peer-reviewed journal of the United States' National Institute of Environmental Health Sciences offers an important vehicle for the dissemination of environmental health information and research findings.

www.ehponline.org

Nutritional Magnesium Association
The mission of the NMA is to disseminate timely and useful information on the subject of nutritional magnesium so as to improve the lives of all people affected by the widespread deficiency of this mineral in our diets and the related health issues associated with this deficiency.

714-605-1100 www.nutritionalmagnesium.org

Hysterectomy Educational Resources and Services

Provides information about the alternatives to and consequences of hysterectomy that are requisite to informed consent.

888-750-4377　www.hersfoundation.com

Our Stolen Future

Provides regular updates about the cutting edge of science related to endocrine disruption.

www.ourstolenfuture.org

PCOS Polycystic Ovary Syndrome

Provides natural health solutions for PCOS, ovarian cysts and polycystic ovaries.

www.ovarian-cysts-pcos.com

Seventh Woman Foundation

Provides education on Wellness through Bioidentical Hormone Replacement Therapies, Nutrition and Life Style Information. *"Hormone Matters for Vital Health"* DVD, and *"Educators Interactive Learning CD"* for the perfect solutions for those who find scientific jargon makes it difficult to get a clear picture of hormone function in the body. Using dynamic visuals these clever tools transcend the complexities.

www.theseventhwoman.com

What Women MUST Know

Dr. Sellman's comprehensive site offering leading-edge information, articles, teleclasses, educational resources and consultation addressing holistic solutions for women's many health concerns.

www.whatwomenmustknow.com

References: Part One

Chapter 1

1. Germaine Greer, *The Change*, Hamish Hamilton, London, 1991
2. John Archer, *Bad Medicine* Simon & Schuster, Australia, 1995, p.217
3. Ibid., p. 192
4. Ibid., p. 211
5. Sandra Coney, *The Menopause Industry*, Spinnifex Press Pty Ltd., Australia, 1991, P. 164-165

Chapter 2

1. Betty Kamen Ph.D.

Chapter 3

1. Marshall, E. "Search For A Killer: Focus Shifts From Fats To Hormones", 1993, *Science* 259: 616-617
2. (a) Dumble, Lynette J., Ph.D., M.Sc., " Odds Against Women with Heart Disease", presented at Health Sharing Women's Forum, Royal College of Surgeons, Melbourne, Victoria, Australia, 14 September, 1995.

   (b) Barrett-Connor, Elisabeth, "Heart Disease in Women", *Fertility and Sterility* (1994), 62(2):1275-132S.

Chapter 4

1. *Menopause News*, Vol. Issue 2 March/April p2
2. *Health Action*, November/December 1985
3. Ibid.

Chapter 5

1. John R. Lee, MD, *What Your Doctor May Not Tell You About Menopause*, Warner Books, New York, 1996 p. 67-68
2. John R. Lee, MD, *Natural Progesterone: The Multiple Role of a Remarkable Hormone*, BLL Publishing, California, 1993, p. 8
3. Ibid., p. 29
4. Lee, op.cit., p. 121
5. Ibid., p. 131
6. Ibid., p. 132

Chapter 6

1. Nancy Beckham, *"Why Women Should Not Take HRT"*,
   Well Being Magazine, No. 67, p. 70

2. Ellen Brown and Lyn Walker, *"Menopause and Estrogen,* Frog Ltd., CA.
   1996, p. 25

3. *Australian Doctor,* August 29, 1997, p. 3

Chapter 8

1. Nancy Beckham, *Menopause - A Positive Approach Using Natural Thera-pies,* Penguin Books Australia Lt. 1995 p. 36-37

2. Ibid., p. 36

3. *British Medial Bulletin,* 1992, 48:458-68

Chapter 9

1. *Newsweek,* March 18, 1996

2. Leslie Kenton, *Passage to Power,* Random House, London, 1995,
   p. 34

3. John Archer -*The Water You Drink, How Safe Is It?,* Pure Water Press,
   1996, p. 34

4. Leslie Kenton, op. cit., p. 32

5. Diane Clorfene-Casten, *"Breast Cancer, Poisons, Profits and Prevention"*,
   Common Courage Press, Maine, 1996, p. 33-34

6. John R. Lee, MD *What Your Doctor May Not Tell You About Menopause,*
   p. 51

7. Ibid., p. 56

8. *Wheel of Hormones,* Lars Mortensen, TV2 Denmark, T.V. Production,
   1995

9. *Green Left Weekly,* June 19, 1996

Chapter 10

1. Lee, op. cit., p. 44

2. *Menopause News,* Vol. Issue 2 March/April p. 2

3. Lee, Jane Lue, "Biomarkers and Prevention", *Cancer Epidemiology,*
   1996, 3:65-70

Chapter 11

1. Lee, op. cit., p. 325
   Menopause, Warner Books, New York, 1996 p. 325

2. *Menopause News,* Vol. Issue 2 March/April p. 1

Chapter 12

1. Kate Neil. *Balancing Hormones Naturally*, ION Press, London, 1994. p. 28
2. John Wilks, *A Consumers Guide To The Pill*, TGB Book, Australia, 1996, p. 81
3. Ibid, pp. 59-60
4. Kate Neil, *Balancing Hormones Naturally*, ION Press, London, 1994. p. 28

Chapter 13

1. *Partners, The AIM News Magazine*, August 1996, p. 22

Chapter 14

1. Lee, op. cit., p. 258
2. Racquel Martin, *The Estrogen Alternative*, Healing Arts Press, Vermont, 1997. p. 109
3. Lee, op. cit. p. 42
4. Christiane Northrup, MD, *Women's Bodies, Women's Wisdom*, Bantam Books, New York p. 158
5. John R. Lee, MD., *Natural Progesterone*, p. 87
6. John R. Lee, MD., op. cit. p. 254
7. Ibid. p. 259
8. Ibid. p. 244
9. John R. Lee, MD., *What Your Doctor May Not Tell You About Menopause*, p. 103
10. Martin, op. cit., p. 43
11. Ibid. p. 230
12. Martin, op. cit., p. 52
13. Lee, op. cit., p. 147
14. Ibid. p. 238
15. Brown and Walker, op. cit., p. 93

Chapter 16

1. Marcus Laux, ND., and Christine Conrad, *Natural Woman, Natural Menopause*, Harper Collins, New York, 1997, p. 79
2. Henry M. Leman, et al, "Reduced Estriol Excretun In Patients With Breast Cancer Prior To Endocrine Therapy", *Journal Of American Medical Association*, 196 (1966): p. 1128-34

Chapter 16 continued

3. Alvin Follingstad, "Estriol For The Forgotten Estrogen", *Journal of American Medical Association*, 239, No.1 (January 2, 1978): p. 29-30

4. Walter E. Stamm and Raul Raz, "A Controlled Trial Of Intravaginal Estriol In Post Menopausal Women With Recurrent Urinary Tract Infections", *Journal Of American Medical Association*, 329, No. 11 (September 9 1993) p. 753-56

Chapter 17

1. D. T. Felson, et al, "The Effect Of Post Menopausal Estrogen Therapy On Bone Density In Elderly Women", *New England Journal Of Medicine*, 329 (1993): pp. 1141-462

2. C. Christensen, et al, "Bone Mass In Post Menopausal Women After The Withdrawal Of Estrogen/Progesterone Therapy", *Lancet*, February 29, 1982: p. 459-61

3. Neil, op. cit., p. 46

4. Kenton, op. cit., p. 19-20

5. Ibid p. 19-20

6. Lee, J. R., Osteoporosis Reversal: The Role of Progesterone. Intern. Clin. Nutr. Rev. 1990, 10:384-391

7. William Regelson, *The Super Hormone Promise*, Simon & Schuster, New York, 1996, p. 186

8. Love, R. R., et. al., "Effects Of Tamoxifen On Women With Breast Cancer", *New England Journal Of Medicine*, 1992, 326: p. 853-6

9. Welton, DC Kempa HCG Post GB Van Stavneren, "A Meta-Analysis Of The Effects For Calcium Intake On Bone Mass In Young, Middle-Aged Females And Males", 1995, WA Nutrition, 125:2802-2813

10. Lee, op. cit., p. 183

11. Love, op. cit., p.97

12. Lee, op. cit., p. 189

13. Myagawa, K., Rosch, J., Stanczk, F. and Hermesmeyer, K., "Medroxy-progesterone Interferes With Ovarian Steroid Protection Against Coronary Vasospasm", *Nature Medicine*, 1997, 3:273-274

14. Sullivan, J. M., Shala Bashau, A., Miller, L. A., Lerner, J. L., and MacBrayer, J. D., "Progestin Enhances Vasoconstrictor Responses In Postmenopausal Women Receiving Estrogen Replacement." *Menopause Journal of North American Menopause Society*, 1995: 2 (4): 193-199

15. Nancy Beckham, op. cit., p. 42-43

16. Lee, op. cit., p. 197

Chapter 17 continued

17. Love, op. cit., p.113

18. *Australian Doctor*, "Breast Risk Double With Long Term HRT", August 29, 1997, p.1

19. Lee, op. cit., p. 208

20. King-Jen Chuang MD, Tigris T.Y. Lee, MD, Gustavo Linares-Cruz, MD, Sabine Fournier, Ph.D. Bruno de Ligneires, MD, "Influences Of Percutaneous Administration Of Estradiol And Progesterone On Human Breast Epithelial Cell Cycle In Vivo. *Fertility and Sterility* April 1995; 63:4 785-791

21. *Journal Of The National Cancer Institute*, 1996: vol 88, 643-49

22. Wilson, P.W.F., Garrison R J, Castelli W P, "Post Menopausal Estrogen Use, Cigarette Smoking And Cardiovascular Morbidity In Women Over 50", The Framingham Study, *New England Journal Of Medicine*, 1985; 313:17, 11038-43

23. Love, op. cit., p.264

24. Beckham, op. cit., p. 48

25. Neil, op. cit., p. 40

26. Clarfene - Casten, op. cit., p. 101

27. Northrup, op. cit., p. 471

28. Kenton op. cit., p. 94

29. Lee, op. cit., p. 220

30. Rodriguez, C., Calle, E. E., Coates, R. J., Miracle-McMahill, H. L., Thun, M. J., and Heath, C. W. Jr., "Estrogen Replacement Therapy And Fatal Ovarian Cancer." *American Journal Of Epidemiology 1995; 141(9) : 828-835*

31. Ellerbrook, J.M., Lee, J.A.H. "Oral contraceptives and malignant melanoma", *Journal of the American Medical Association* 1968; 206:649

32. *The Walnut Creek Contraceptive Drug Study* Vol III, NIH Pub. 1986 and including Beral,V., Ramcharan, S., Faris, R., "Malignant Melanoma And Oral Contraceptive Use Among Women In California." p 247-52.

33 Beral, V., Evans S., Shaw, H., Milton, G., "Oral Contraceptive Use And Malignant Melanoma In Australia." *British Journal of Cancer,* 1984; 50:681-85

34. Love. op. cit. p. 134

35. Paganini-Hill, A., and Henderson, V.W. "Estrogen deficiency and risk of Alzheimer's disease in women." American Journal of Epidemiology 1994;1140(3):256-2261

36. Brown and Walker, op. cit. p. xiv

37. Love. op. cit. p. 136

Chapter 18

1. Lee, op. cit., p. 79
2. The Burton Goldberg Group, *Alternative Medicine*, Future Medicine Publishing, Inc., Puyallup, Washington, 1993, p. 737
3. Martin, op. cit. p. 118-119

Chapter 20

1. *The Sunday Telegraph*, London, May 12, 1996

Dr. Sherrill Sellman, N.D.

Heroine for Natural Hormone Health

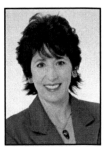

Dr. Sherrill Sellman, a Naturopathic Doctor and Board Certified in Integrative Medicine, is a leading voice in women's holistic health and wellness. She is internationally respected as a dynamic lecturer, authoritative writer and health journalist assisting women to access truthful information and safe holistic solutions regarding the many aspects of their hormonal health and wellbeing.

Dr. Sellman is also a best selling author, senior editor for *TotalHealth Magazine*, psychotherapist, and president of WomanWise International, a health consulting company.

Through her books, articles, lectures and personal consultations, Dr. Sellman has assisted women globally to achieve greater health. She is a sought-after keynote speaker and educator facilitating classes, seminars and lectures in the US, Canada, Ireland, England, Australia and New Zealand. In addition, she has conducted corporate trainings on stress management, personal development and women's wellness.

Dr. Sellman also hosts a weekly internet radio show with respected health experts called, "What Women MUST Know" (www.progressiveradionetwork.com) empowering women with truthful information and in-depth, candid conversations regarding their bodies, hormones and pertinent life issues. All her shows are archived and can be accessed at any time.

Dr. Sellman is available for personal consultations with women via the phone or Skype!

As a passionate, inspiring and powerful voice for the empowerment and health of women of all ages, Dr. Sellman has truly found her mission in life.

For more information about Dr. Sellman's programs, free articles and teleclasses, consulting services or lecture schedule, please visit www.whatwomenmustknow.com or email golight@earthlink.net.

Author of :

Hormone Heresy:
What Women MUST Know About Their Hormones
What Women MUST Know to Protect Their Daughters
From Breast Cancer
Salba, The Return of the Ancient Seed

Index

A

Acne 24, 39, 41, 45, 73, 89, 206, 331

Adrenal glands 16, 27, 28, 33, 78, 163, 208, 210

Aeron Life Cycle Laboratory 56

Alcohol 83, 88, 111, 213, 214, 217, 250, 305, 306

Allergies 34, 64, 78, 180, 183, 200, 203, 204, 210, 269, 290

Alzheimer's disease 107, 122

Amenorrhoea 41

Androgens 89

Anovulatory cycles 30-33, 66, 81, 82, 110, 115
    and premenopause syndrome testing of 12

Armour 207

Arthritis 26, 78, 183, 242, 277
    and DES 26

Auto immune 34, 79

Auto immune disorders 34, 79

B

Batmanchelidj, Dr. 183

Beckham, Nancy 39, 47, 64, 114, 338, 340

Beta-carotene 116

Bioflavonoids 176, 309

Bio-identical Hormone Replacement Therapy (BHRT) 203

Birth defects 39, 40

Bloating 69, 87, 141, 142, 148, 203, 205, 211

Blood clots 64, 70, 109, 113, 147, 205

Blood serum testing 60

Blood sugar 21, 33, 35, 76, 83, 179

Blood sugar control 21, 35

Bone formation 31, 36, 109, 111

Bone mineral density 73

Boron 175

Bounous, Dr. Gustavo 277

Brain 11, 12, 14, 16, 40, 50, 53, 67, 77, 83, 87, 88, 112, 123, 163, 179, 183, 213, 232, 240, 247-249, 289, 292, 299, 302
    and progesterone 11, 77
    and hypothalamus 14
    and PMS 87
    and sex hormones 50, 88

Brain function 40, 88, 179, 183, 292

Breast cancer 20, 24, 29, 33, 36, 43, 51, 52, 56, 64-66, 76, 97, 103, 104, 111, 116-120, 122-124, 149, 151, 177, 183, 184, 187, 194, 227, 232, 243-245, 248, 264, 290, 299-302, 316, 335

Breast milk 40, 51, 52

Benefits 84, 185

Brown, Susan E., PhD 234

Bruce Ettinger, Dr. 233

C

Caffeine 83, 111, 179

Calcium 107, 108, 111, 112, 176, 179, 180, 232, 235-237, 263, 291, 293, 294, 320, 321, 333

Candida 70, 79, 204, 205, 295, 308

Cardiovascular disease 20, 45, 107, 112-116, 242, 264, 279

Castration 97, 126, 127, 227

Cervical cancer 25, 64, 121

Chocolate 83, 87, 179, 307

Cholesterol 27, 43, 73, 88, 113, 115, 205, 206, 234, 263, 266, 283, 317, 326
    and dyslipidemia 115

Chronic fatigue 36, 137, 141, 269, 271, 279

Chronic Fatigue Syndrome 209, 290

Coffee Enema Recipe 220

Colburn, Theo 50

Colditz 8, 116, 117

Corpus luteum 86

Corticosteroids 28, 75, 78, 125

Cortisol 31, 209, 213, 248, 253, 302, 303, 329

Cortisone 76, 78, 79, 111

Creative Menopause
and Farida Sharan 163

Crohn's disease 279

D

Dairy products 51, 111, 180, 217, 232, 236

Dalton, Dr. Katherina 72

Dehydration 183, 184, 306

Depo-Provera 39, 42, 63, 64

Depression 21, 34, 39, 41, 47, 48, 55, 56, 64, 69, 73-75, 84, 85, 87, 89, 97, 99, 119, 143, 145, 179, 185, 200, 203, 205, 206, 210-214, 226, 227, 248, 250, 287, 302
and post partum 85
and tamoxifen 119

DES 23, 24, 26

Diabetes 83, 179

Diet 18, 31, 34, 65, 66, 74, 81, 82, 84, 90, 98, 103-105, 108, 112, 126, 145, 151, 170, 175, 177, 204, 205, 207, 213, 221, 236, 237, 254, 255, 258, 261, 264, 278, 281, 289, 303, 305
and heart disease 84
and PMS 74

Diethylstilbestrol 23

Dumanoski, Dianne
and Xeno estrogens 50

Dumble, Dr. Lynnette 7, 20, 337

Duphaston 39

E

Eczema 200, 206, 325

Eggs 11, 14, 16, 163, 207, 223, 261

EMR 297, 298, 300-304

Endometrial cancer 7, 21, 35, 57, 76, 97, 109, 121

Endometrial hyperplasia 225

Endometriosis 21, 29, 34, 53, 79-81, 97, 180, 206, 227, 242, 264, 269, 290

Essential fatty acids 64, 126, 175, 177, 180, 214

Estradiol 12, 27, 47, 56, 61, 104, 115, 118-121, 125, 126, 177, 241, 242, 329

Estriol 27, 91, 96, 98, 104, 105, 120, 242, 245

Estrogen 1-15, 19-21, 23, 24, 26-34, 36, 37, 39, 41-43, 45, 47-52, 55-57, 59, 60, 63, 65, 66, 71, 73-84, 86-91, 94-100, 103-105, 108-111, 113-126, 131, 132, 137-139, 142, 143, 145, 149, 150, 162, 176, 177, 203-207, 211-213, 215-217, 220, 223, 225, 227, 228, 232, 237, 241-245, 264, 283-285, 298, 299-301, 328

Estrogen Deficiency 55, 74, 91

Estrogen Dominance 27, 29, 32, 34, 36, 39, 49, 56, 65, 74, 79, 81, 82, 87, 90, 99, 117, 121, 131, 142, 145

Estrogens
natural 103

Estrone 27, 56, 104, 116, 119, 120, 121, 241, 242

Exercise 9, 34, 66, 84, 98, 111, 112, 116, 129, 136, 186-188, 214, 217, 236, 237, 257, 279, 281

F

Fallopian tube 12

Fatigue 32, 33, 36, 42, 45, 87, 99, 137, 141, 150, 179, 203, 205, 206, 209, 211, 213, 225, 269, 271, 279, 312, 319

Fertility 27, 67, 68, 118, 216, 239-242, 246, 263, 285, 302, 337, 341

Fibrocystic breasts 73, 99, 139, 264

Fibroids 21, 29, 35, 36, 81, 97, 100, 180, 206, 215-218, 220, 221, 225, 227, 242, 264, 310
    Reason for hysterectomies 97

Fibromyalgia 78, 137, 139

Fish 50, 177, 178, 207, 285, 286, 307, 309-316
    hermaphroditic 50

Fluoride 111, 207

Follicles 11, 13-16, 33, 50, 84, 86, 89, 163, 241
    burnout 50, 84
    depletion 163

Follicle stimulating hormone (FSH) 12, 86, 165

Follicular phase 121, 160

Follicular stage 13

Follingstad, Dr. A. H. 104

G

Gardasil 199

Glutathione 275-281, 322, 332

Goddess 157, 158, 162

Grains 84, 90, 145, 175, 180, 208, 214, 261, 305, 306

Greer, Germaine 2, 55, 337

H

Hair loss 64, 73, 82, 203, 225

Hargraves, Dr. Joel T. 88

Harvard Medical School 24

Hashimoto 79

HCG 254-258, 326, 340

Herbicides 33, 49, 175, 291

Homeopathy 71

Hormone addiction 47

Hormone balance 90, 183, 213, 264, 303, 317

Hormone Replacement Therapy 5, 7, 47, 55, 79, 94, 110, 132, 203

Hot flashes 47, 55, 61, 73-75, 83, 84, 96, 98, 103, 119, 140, 143-145, 148, 176, 177, 186, 187, 203, 209, 242, 312, 327
    frequency of 84
    reduction of 84
    symptoms of 96

Hot flushes 47, 55, 73, 75, 83, 98, 103, 176

HRT 7-9, 11, 21, 29, 34, 39, 42, 47, 48, 55, 59, 74, 95, 98, 105, 107, 109, 112, 113, 118, 122, 136-145, 149-151, 203, 204, 206, 212, 213, 236, 254, 338, 341

Hypertension 29, 37, 73, 82, 113, 214

Hypoglycemia 21, 35, 70, 205

Hypothalamus 12, 15, 83, 165

Hypothyroidism 34, 73, 83, 90, 200, 205-208, 213, 216, 220, 290

Hysterectomies 96

Hysterectomy 80, 81, 95-97, 105, 108, 115, 121, 139, 215, 216, 221, 223-229, 336

Hysterectomy Hoax 96

I

Infertility 21, 29, 35, 52, 64, 84, 96, 206, 248

Inquisition 2, 3, 158

Insomnia 39, 41, 47, 126, 141, 143, 200, 203, 205, 210-214, 225, 247, 287, 312
    and Provera 41

Intracellular 29, 82, 87, 277, 280

Intracellular hypoxia 29

J

Johns Hopkins
    private Ob/Gyn Clinic 117

Journal of American Medical Association 104

K

Kamen, Betty 13

Kenton, Leslie 8, 37, 132, 338, 340, 341

Kidney 179, 183, 264

L

Lanksy, Dr. Ephraim 242

Lauersen, Dr. Neil 43, 87

Lee, Dr. John R. 8, 21, 29, 31-33, 45, 56, 66, 68, 72-74, 77-82, 84, 85, 87, 89, 90, 94, 96, 98, 100, 107, 113-115, 127, 132, 337-342

Lemon, Dr. H.M. 104

Libido 14, 29, 69, 75, 87, 88-90, 127, 137, 139, 146, 148, 211, 214, 226, 245, 290, 327

Liver detoxification 218

Lou Gehrig's Disease 279

Love, Dr. Susan 60, 112, 119

Low libido 88, 90, 211

L-theanine 248-250

Lupus 26, 34, 79

Luteal phase 13, 84, 87, 120, 160, 161

Luteinizing hormone (LH) 12, 86

M

MaxGXL 322

Mead, Margaret 18

Meditation 165, 189, 190, 214

Medroxyprogesterone 40

Menopause 2, 3, 6, 9, 15, 20, 24-57, 32, 47, 64, 88, 98, 162, 163, 169, 196, 204, 241, 312, 337-340

Menopause industry 3, 337

Menstrual cycle 94
    and progesterone 28
    irregular 27

Methyl-testosterone 45

Meyers, John Peterson
    xeno estrogens 50

Milk 40, 180

Miscarriage 15, 23-25, 85, 139, 290

Multiple Sclerosis 279

Myelin 78

N

Natural progesterone 31, 34, 36-40, 43, 45, 68, 71-75, 77, 78, 80-82, 84, 86-90, 93, 94, 95-101, 105, 108, 111, 113, 120, 125, 127, 139, 142, 145, 147, 148, 150, 151, 214, 216, 236, 328
    and arthritis 79
    and endometrial cancer 37
    and fibrocystic breast 36
    and fibroids 36, 81
    benefits of 77
    bone mineral density 73
    increased levels 31
    loss of pregnancy 84
    side effects 75
    treating endometriosis 80
    vaginal dryness and hot flashes 73
    vs. progestins 39

New England Journal of Medicine 7, 24, 104, 110, 114

Nonylphenols 33, 53, 80

Norplant 39, 42, 63, 64

Northrup 80, 339

O

Oils 178

Oophorectomy 4, 97

Oral contraceptives 5, 19, 63, 82, 113, 122, 136

Organic produce 54

Osteoblasts 31, 36, 108, 232, 233

Osteoclasts 108, 109, 232, 233

Osteonecrosis 235

Osteoporosis 7, 20, 29, 31, 33-36, 55, 56, 70, 72, 73, 76, 97, 99, 107-112, 127, 137, 141, 181, 199, 203, 205, 207, 224, 229, 231-237, 244, 248, 340
    bone loss tests 99

Ovarian cancer 6, 121, 224, 244, 341

Ovarian cysts 29, 206, 218, 225, 264, 336

Ovaries 4, 5, 11-16, 27, 28, 33, 36, 37, 50, 59, 60, 66, 67, 70, 71, 84-86, 89, 97, 108, 117, 120, 162, 163, 169, 177, 220, 223, 224, 227, 229, 241, 336

Ovulation 12-14, 30, 56, 66, 68, 82, 84-86, 89, 117, 146, 160, 211

P

PeakImmune4 271-274, 319

Peat, Ray PhD 72

Perimenopausal 18, 34, 99, 100, 121, 163, 200, 214, 242

Perimenopause 29, 74, 211, 212, 328

Petrochemicals 49

Physicians' Desk Reference 40, 113

Physicians' Desk Reference (PDR) 40

Phytoestrogens 103

Pill 19, 20, 63-70, 90, 113, 122, 136, 144-148, 195, 196, 199, 206, 216, 339

Pituitary 12, 15, 41, 165, 207, 220

PMS 29, 30, 35, 43, 72-74, 87, 88, 101, 146, 147, 159, 161, 180, 206, 210-212, 242, 248, 250, 264

Pomegranate 91, 239-244, 246, 311, 313, 316, 317 320, 325, 327, 334

Post menopause 55

Post natal depression 84

Primulut 39, 40, 149

Prior, Dr. Jerilynn 32, 34, 55, 57, 110, 114, 212

Progesterone 7, 13-15, 27-34, 36, 37, 39, 40, 43, 45, 49, 56, 59, 63, 67, 68, 71, 86-90, 93, 94-101, 104, 105, 108, 109-113, 115-118, 120, 125-127, 132, 139, 142, 145, 147, 148, 150, 151, 162, 204, 207, 209, 211, 212, 214, 216, 223, 227, 236, 242, 298, 309, 311-316, 327-329, 337, 339-341

Progesterone deficiency 29-31, 36, 72, 74, 75, 77, 78, 81, 84, 85, 88-90, 110-112, 115, 118, 204, 212

Progestins 3, 19, 39, 40, 42, 121
   blocking progesterone 40
   intensify PMS 43

Prostacyclin 17, 226

Prostate cancer 24, 53, 57, 125, 126, 284, 300

Provera 39, 40, 42, 63, 64, 94, 114, 137, 138, 140
   potential side effect 40

Puberty 11, 12, 27, 65, 66, 285, 290

R

Radiation 207

Robbins, John 96

S

Saliva testing 56, 60, 126, 212

Scientific American 109

Simeons, Dr. 10, 56, 60, 126, 212, 255-259

Skakkebeak, Neils 52

Skin problems 56, 60, 89, 126, 212

Smoking 56, 60, 113, 116, 126, 212

Soybeans 56, 60, 126, 176, 212

Stress 28-34, 42, 65, 75, 78, 83-85, 88, 98, 116, 126, 129, 143, 145, 179, 183-185, 189, 204, 207, 209, 210, 213, 214, 216, 221, 224, 247-250, 253, 254, 265, 269, 276, 277, 279, 298, 299, 302, 303, 315, 333
   and adrenal exhaustion 78
   and anovulatory cycles 31
   and corticosteroids 28
   and estrogen dominance 29
   and fight or flight 31
   and heart disease 116
   and hormonal imbalances 33
   and hormone levels 32
   and integrated therapies 129
   and proper breathing 185
   and refined sugar 179
   and lessening 116

Sugar 21, 28, 33, 35, 47, 70, 76, 83, 111, 145, 179, 184, 205, 209, 213, 214, 217, 254, 258, 263, 266, 305, 306, 317, 320, 326, 330, 331
    and bone density 111
    and coronary disease 116
    and placebos 47

Sugar pills 47, 56, 60, 126, 212

Suntheanine 56, 60, 126, 212, 249, 250, 251

Surwit, Dr. Earl 91, 245

Susan, Dr. Love 14

Synthroid 56, 60, 126, 207, 212

T

Tamoxifen 62, 104, 111
    and bone loss 119
    and breast cancer 119

Testes 28, 33, 125

Testicular cancer 26

Testosterone 28, 45, 50, 75-78, 89, 125,-127, 137, 149, 150, 223, 298, 301, 329
    and long-term safety 45

The Change 2, 337

Thrush 69, 70

Thyroid deficiency 69, 89

Tofu 89, 103, 112, 177

Total Health Magazine 89, 200

Total Silver 293-295

Type 2 Diabetes 266

U

Ultimate Fat Loss 254, 326

Unopposed estrogen 7, 89

Uterine lining 14, 89

Uterus 4, 11-15, 17, 25, 27, 73, 75, 79, 80, 88, 96, 97, 103, 108, 117, 125, 138, 218, 221-227, 231
    effects of phytoestrogens 103
    removal of 96

V

Vitamins 89, 116, 179, 180, 181

Vuksan, Vladimir 262, 265, 266

W

Weight bearing exercise 89, 111, 112, 188

Weight gain 30, 33, 36, 87, 90, 100, 126, 137, 147, 150, 179, 200, 203, 206, 209, 211, 213, 225, 227, 253, 254

Weight loss 28, 253, 254, 256-259, 266, 272, 326

West, Dr. Stanley 96

Westhroid 89, 207

Wild yam 71, 72, 89, 93

Wilson, Dr. Robert 5

Wyeth-Ayerst Laboratories 6

X

Xeno estrogens 85, 89

Y

Yeast infection 70, 89

Z

Zava 56, 89

Zinc 21, 35, 64, 76, 207, 210, 213, 263, 321, 324